New Nurse? How to Get, Keep and LOVE Your First Job!

Caroline Porter Thomas

PRAISE for

Caroline and EmpoweRN!

"Your writing touches the core of those who seek to be in this field. I am so blessed to have come across your work and I believe it is not by chance. You are an old soul, Caroline. You are doing exactly what you have been called to do and the nursing field needs more people like you who are doing the right things for the right reasons. I appreciate your honesty and humility and above all your desire to be of help. I wish you all the best and again, thank you for doing what you do."

- Sonia Tan

"I just came across your Youtube videos and watched every single one of them! They were all amazing.. I start nursing school in about a week, I am very excited. I look forward to more videos and inspiration from you!"

- Ashley Wyers Benson

"I appreciate all of your help so much. It's so comforting to know that there are people like you who make it their personal mission to assist nursing students - it's very much needed, as this is definitely the most challenging school experience that I've ever had to go through. Not only is there so much material to cover in such a small amount of time, along with a new type of "critical thinking" question format to get use to, but on top of it all, it's finding the motivation to continue on. I've

Caroline Porter Thomas

found that your videos did just that - it gave me the
motivation I needed to keep going; that second wind. For
that, I truly can't thank you enough. Thank you for all you
do and for being so generous with your knowledge and
experience with all of us. It's an honor and a gift to receive
tips from an honors nursing student and RN. All the best to
you and much love to you as well :o)"

- Bernadette Zapata

"Thanks a bunch Caroline! I will always be in
touch. I admire your heart to help us Nursing Students."

- Kehinde Tayewo

"I have been watching your videos for a really long time
and I earned a lot from your experiences and methods. I
just want to thank you for everything your doing. You are
realy heping so many people that struggle with so much in
order to be a professional nurse and make their dreams
come true. Really, thank you."

- Dalal Al-Mutairi from Saudi Arabia

"I love watching your Youtube channel EmpoweRN,
You inspire me all the time!"

- Susan Leyshon

"I wanted to let you know how much I have
enjoyed reading your first book! Thank you for writing
How To Succeed In Nursing School and taking the time to
video your blog entries too! Thanks for all the helpful tips!

I'm already using the 7 day challenge for making the list the night before (using the format you gave in your book!). I look forward to reading your second book once I have RN behind my name."

- Sheena from Southern California

"Thank you so much for your prompt reply and great tips :) I am so excited, started your tips today. I checked out 2 more nclex style question books like you mentioned from Phoenix college lib. Awesome ! Thanks again and I am looking forward to better grades :) yay! And I will do your 20 workouts if nothing else. Everyday will add up. And I saw your eating for energy during school tips, you look amazing so I know it works.. okay thanks again for sharing your tips to the world :)"

- Brenda Armenta

Caroline Porter Thomas

New Nurse? How to Get, Keep and LOVE Your First Job!

Disclaimer

Publishing information: EmpoweRN Inc.

For information about special discounts for bulk purposes, please contact Caroline directly at (305) 975-5946 or Caroline@EmpoweRN.com. She is also available to speak at your institution.

Manufactured in the United States of America

ISBN-13: 978-1484177525

ISBN-10: 1484177525

Caroline Porter Thomas

New Nurse?

How to Get, Keep and LOVE Your First Nursing Job!

Caroline Porter Thomas, BSN, RN

Caroline Porter Thomas

Acknowledgments

This book is dedicated to my subscribers and fans on Youtube, Twitter and Facebook via: EmpoweRN. Through this vessel, you all have opened your hearts, minds and souls to me. I am always amazed at how loving, generous, vulnerable and supportive you are with my videos, tweets, post and emails. Thank you for giving me this exciting and life transforming purpose. Without all of your love and support my dream of EmpoweRN would not be possible.

I look forward to an exciting future with you; one that will help us all live in a reverent, joyful, service mentality. As we all grow and become better and better nurses we will raise the standards of what compassionate and loving care is.

This book is also dedicated to the nurses who have shown me exactly how to deliver a loving touch. I learn ever day from my fellow co-workers who I am blessed to work with.

And of course, I wouldn' t be anywhere without my amazing and loving husband Emmanuel. Your big dreams, dedication to your purpose, belief and practice in consistent hard work is a great model for me to follow. I am so grateful that I get to share my life with you. I love you and I see an exciting future with you!

Caroline Porter Thomas

New Nurse?

How to Get, Keep and LOVE Your First Nursing Job!

Chapters:

Caroline Porter Thomas

Foreword

It was my second year of college. I entered the Chemistry 2 classroom and totally freaked out. I had barely gotten a B in Chemistry 1 and now had moved from Florida to North Carolina to a new school. I was in a completely different class with a different instructor and classmates. Not even the book was the same... I had no idea how I was going to pass. But I knew that even passing wouldn't be enough! I had to get an A!
I was constantly reminding myself of how competitive it was to gain acceptance into nursing school.

I sat in the front of the classroom to hopefully surround myself with people who would be enthusiastic and know what they were doing. Throughout the entire first hour of class, the instructor asked a few review questions. My heart sank as the word "Review" came before ideas, concepts and problems that my former instructor had not put as much emphasis on.

There was one classmate, however, who was faster at shouting out the answer than anyone else. He caught my attention. After class, I went over and talked to him. He completed Chemistry 1 with the same instructor last semester and received an A. That was all I needed to hear. "Will you tutor me?" I asked. He agreed after we spoke with the instructor, and she also thought it would be a good idea.

The next few months were challenging. Nothing came easily for me. I struggled with every single concept and problem. I would see my tutor not even study and hang out with friends the night before tests and pass with A's. Frustration did not even begin to describe my feeling.

One day, however, I finally made my first A on a test. My hard work was starting to pay off. I had developed excellent study habits and, from then on, received A's much more often. Then something strange happened.

One Monday, I got a test back from my instructor. "Oh, yay, a 94%," I said happily. My tutor peered at me. "I got 89%," he replied. I stared at him, feeling awkward and bad for him.

Looking back on this hard lesson, I realized that learning from other people is great way to get ahead. When you learn from others, no matter how smart they are, you still bring to the table your "sometimes limited" but useful knowledge. This knowledge expands upon what is being taught to you.

My father once said that the best hope you can have for your children is that you teach them to be better than you.

I'm not sure my Chemistry tutor shared the same feeling. But that is my intention with this book. I've been a nurse for five years. I want to help you learn from my successes and mistakes, so you can soar to levels of happiness you never imagined possible. Remember, no matter how lost you can feel on your first job, you bring valuable experiences, knowledge and, most importantly, your beautiful presence.

I truly hope one day that I meet you face to face, and we can talk about how much you love your life as a nurse.

With love,
Caroline Porter Thomas
Caroline@EmpoweRN.com

Caroline Porter Thomas

Chapter 1

Get the Interview

"Everything you want should be yours: the type of work you want; the relationships you need; the social, mental, and aesthetic stimulation that will make you happy and fulfilled; the money you require for the lifestyle that is appropriate to you; and any requirement that you may (or may not) have for achievement of service to others. If you don't aim for it all, you'll never get it all. To aim for it requires that you know what you want."
-Richard Koch

I was on top of the world. I had just married the love of my life and was moving to be with him at his home in Bethesda, Maryland. I had been working as a nurse for two years at a small hospital in the middle of nowhere, Sanford, NC. Man, I loved that hospital. It was small, beautiful and full of smiling faces I knew well and still miss today.

I started there as a graduate and worked through different roles on the main Tele/Med-Surg floor. I remember my interview with the director, Ms. Tysinger. "Call me Liz," she said as I shook her hand and we sat down. She asked me a few questions, and it was so easy to talk to her. She had a warm, sweet spirit and I instantly loved her.

Those few questions were all she asked. Then she explained how things went on the unit. I felt as though she hoped I would choose that hospital and her unit. Directly after that, I interviewed for a similar unit, one floor below. The interview went fine, but I didn't feel the connection with the director and ultimately chose to work with Liz.

This interview experience was so awesome that, when I moved from North Carolina to Maryland, I expected more of the same. And now I had two years of valuable experience! I was sure to be a shoe in.

I found the top two hospitals that were very close to me and spent all of my time and attention applying to them. Two weeks went by without a call. I'm not the type of person who likes to be unemployed, so these were some of the longest two weeks of my life. No phone call. What was going on?

I figured they must need to put a face to the application. I dressed in my best and visited the human resources departments. I was greeted by unpleasant faces and told there was no one I could talk to and I just had to wait for a call.

The calls never came.

Completely flustered, I began to apply to absolutely every hospital, home health agency, and doctor's office accepting registered nurse applicants. I spent five to six hours a day filling out application after application. I also spent countless hours with my husband reviewing my resume. Finally, another two weeks went by and then... a few calls and emails started to come.

I'm telling you my story as a nurse with experience. I know that for new graduates, especially those with no hospital experience, the job market nowadays can be more challenging even than what I experienced. However, new graduates do get hired all the time, on every type of unit -- Med/Surg, of course, but also ICUs, Labor and Delivery units and even trauma ICUs.

Liz asked me to be a precept with my first new graduate when I had just over six months of experience. Boy, was I scared, but she believed in me, so I did it. One of the best things about being a preceptor, though, was attending an invaluable class to understand my role better.

I learned how much time, energy and effort was given to new graduates. Not just mine as a preceptor, but also that of the hospital and unit directors. I learned that it takes almost $40,000 to train a new graduate. And that was in North Carolina where the nursing salary is much less than many states. I imagine in other states this number could go up to $55,000 easily. That day I understood why hiring a new graduate was a big deal.

Imagine being a unit director of a Med/Surg unit. You have a budget that will support three new graduates for this year. You have eight wonderful choices of smart, eager and fresh applicants.

However, one of them expressed how she just wanted to get her feet wet in Med/Surg but ultimately saw herself working in the ICU.

Basically, that nurse is saying that after you spend your $40,000 on me, I am going to leave you after a year. I clearly understood why many hospitals require new graduates to sign a two-year contract. Two years, by the way, is what I believe it takes to be safe in an RN position these days.

Understanding the challenges that hospitals and directors face, you must look at each interview as if you are asking for at least $40,000.

The Application Process

Before you get the interview, you have to get the call. And to get the call you must fill out the application perfectly, which is time consuming, and make sure that resume is polished.

I used to believe the resume wasn't a big deal. I mean, all of the information on the resume is duplicated on the application. So one time I neglected to update it. Then I got a call from a prospective director who was interested in me, but who said the resume indicated I wasn't currently working. Ooops. I had to explain that my resume wasn't correct and that I was working. Keep your resume updated!

I don't believe the template used for your resume matters. If you search Google images for resume, you'll see a number of different formats. Just make sure everything is clean, concise and error-free. I've been asked if I use an image of myself and personally I have not. I don't see anything wrong with doing so, though.

When it comes to your references, be selective. You may need to include past managers and directors of other units, if this isn't your first nursing job. Make sure you either left on good terms or try somehow to ask if they wouldn't mind putting in a good word for you as you apply for jobs. The key is to always make sure the people who are being called are prepared.

I have been asked by a number of people to be a reference for them, and I definitely spend time preparing myself for the call that may come. Also, at the end of the resume you can add "additional references." Here is your opportunity to add the assistant director who absolutely loved you and is a great talker, or that co-worker who was so awesome to work with.

As I said, always ask the individuals if they wouldn't mind being a reference for you. Listen to their responses carefully since this is your livelihood that you are talking about. For example, I was looking for some awesome "additional references," people who liked me and loved to talk about how great I was.

So I asked two different people from the same department to see who sounded the best when asked the question. The first was a guy who really surprised me. So my question was this: "Hi, blank, I'm applying to jobs and was wondering if you could put in a good word for me by being a reference." His response was this. "All I can say is the dates that you worked here and if anyone complained about you." Really? Unfortunately, because of lawsuits, many businesses have taken that approach to requests for references.

Needless to say, I didn't like that response. So I asked his co-worker the same question. And this was her response. "Caroline, I would be honored to be a reference for you. You are one of the best nurses we have, and we are so sorry to see you go. I was at a meeting yesterday and I had four directors saying how great you were!" Guess who I used as my additional, professional reference.

When you ask, don't take the responses personally. I could have been hurt by the first person I asked. But, maybe he is not the type of person who likes being asked these types of questions, or maybe he had too many calls already for references or maybe he just felt as if he didn't know me well enough. Just ask different people until you find someone who is willing to show the side of you that you want to present to your future employer.

The last step to get the interview is to apply like crazy everywhere. You're doing this for two reasons. The first, of course, is to get a job, but the second is for the valuable interview experience. The next chapter is dedicated to the actual interview so stay tuned, but realize that it is a very awkward experience if you are not prepared.

I, too, would love to work at the hospital that has the best reputation and is also 5 minutes away from me. However, you must apply to every single hospital within an hour drive from your location. As a new graduate it is more challenging for you to get hired. You are a big risk for the hospital to take on. In order to get a job, you may have to take your first job a little farther away, and you may have to take the 7 p.m. to 7 a.m. shift.

For my first job, I rotated between three weeks of day shifts and then three weeks of night shifts for over a year. Do what you have to do to get experience. By the way, I recommend rotating as opposed to strictly night shift or day shift because it gives you a good overall view of how that unit operates. Also, you get to see what both shifts are like so in the future you can decide if you want to do strictly day or night shifts when the positions become available.

When I moved to Maryland, I spent an entire month finding places to apply and filling out applications. You will most likely have to do the same. It may take awhile before you even get your first phone call. Remember, it took me two weeks before I got my first response. My first interview was almost one month later, and I didn't start working for almost two months.

Just keep applying and eventually, you'll get responses. Fill out every single application perfectly and carefully. Think over every single word carefully. For the resume, look at it and say to yourself: Does this person deserve $40,000? If not, make it better. Give it your all and keep at it. If you do, you'll get those phone calls soon.

Also, as a last point, if you're still a nursing student and you have some time left, apply as a volunteer on a unit where you would be interested in working. Or see if you can work as a Nursing Assistant (if you have the credential). The first thing they will tell you when they find out you are in nursing school is that this will not increase your chances of getting hired.

But seriously, how can it not? I guess if you're really bad and lazy... but I could hardly see that being the case. If directors have 20 applications in front of them and they see a name they recognize and they happen to like you... Believe me, it does help but, of course, can't guarantee success. Keep in mind that volunteering in your field will look good on your resume. Even if that director can't offer you a job, maybe you could use her as a reference.

Chapter 2

Ace the Interview

"Don't waste your life in doubts and fears: spend yourself on the work before you, well assured that the right performance of this hour's duties will be the best preparation for the hours or ages that follow it." – Ralph Waldo Emerson

I walked through the hallway past the front desk trying to navigate myself through to the Human Resources department. I felt really good. Finally, to be back in a hospital! It had been a month since I moved to Maryland, and I was now getting regular calls and scheduled interviews from all of the applications that I placed. This was the first and it was at a really good hospital in Baltimore Maryland.

I didn't prepare too much. I had two years of relevant experience for the job I applied for. They practically wouldn't have to train me, just a week or two to have someone show me where things were. I would start work in no time, I figured.

As I approached the department, I looked down at my phone. 10:55. Perfect timing, I thought. It was a good idea to leave really early as parking was an issue and it gave me time to actually find the department. I was welcomed by stone-cold faces once again in the HR department. I wonder if this is a requirement for the job in the state of Maryland?

"Fill this out and then have a seat over there," the HR secretary instructed. As I sat down, I browsed through the papers and there were three whole pages of additional questions, all the same questions I had already answered on the application. Luckily, I learned from experience that you always bring all of your documents with you.

So I pulled out my envelope that contained my application information. In this envelope, I also have my birth certificate, my passport (for additional identification), my degree, my social security card, my shot record and all of my other health documents, my Basic Life Support (BLS) card, my Advanced Cardiac Life Support (ACLS) card, everything. You name it, it's in there.

Filling out all of the information took me literally 30 minutes, after which I was led into a room with three other people. All appeared to be waiting for their interviews, as well. "Were they all interviewing for the same position?" I wondered. As I spoke with a few, one person was indeed interviewing for the exact same position. I never felt like I had competition for a job interview, but now I did.

My nerves were really playing a number on me. I kept comparing myself to the other person interviewing for the position. I didn't even know her but somehow I was thinking she was a better candidate. What was I doing here and, man, wouldn't it be great just to go back to my hospital in North Carolina, where everyone was so warm and welcoming?

"It is time to grow, Caroline," I told myself. I thought that even if I don't get hired, I have two other interviews for different hospitals already scheduled. This will be a good experience so that I will be better prepared for the next interviews. At that point, I was able to take a nice deep breath and relax a little.

Until I heard her come down the hall. Click, click, click was an obnoxious sound that echoed, seeming to put everyone on edge. Then she entered the room. She wore a royal blue business suit with a straight skirt, nude tights and very pointy shoes. Her hair was light brunette and wrapped up into a tight bun on the top of her head. The only makeup she wore was eyeliner on the watermark of her eye, which made her cold blue eyes stand out. "Ms. Thomas?" she said as she looked at all of the applicants.

She took me for what seemed to be a 5-minute walk, passing three different elevators, the cafeteria and all kinds of winding hallways. When we finally approached her office, all I could think about was how I was going to get back home. She must have read my mind because the first thing was that it looked more confusing than it really was.

Once in her office, she motioned for me to have a seat on the opposite end of her desk. She didn't waste any time and began asking questions immediately. "So, Caroline, tell me about yourself."

Right then I knew that this was going to be hard. In my opinion, this is the most difficult question to ask someone on an interview. The question is just so broad. Do they want to hear about your work history, your personality, your successes?

I don't even remember what I said. I do know that there were a lot of umm's and likes to fill space. It seemed like when she had enough, she asked me the next question. "What do you know about our organization?" Ok, really.

"I know that you advertised an opening in my specialty…" I didn't say that, but that is what I was thinking. This is a hospital, and aren't they all about the same?

"Why do you want to work for us?" and then she finished with, "Why should we hire you?" Finally, it was over. She stood up, thanked me for my time as I did the same to her. It took me 20 minutes to reach the front of the hospital. For two reasons, the first being that I was feeling so bad and confused that I was having a hard time focusing and the second was because she took me down so many winding hallways and different floors, I was completely lost.

No one could have ever given me a greater gift. Seriously, I now knew what I needed to do to ace the interviews in the coming weeks. Think about it. Had I not filled out a million applications, I would not have had this experience and might have done poorly at a hospital that I was more interested in.

So the first thing I did when I got home was Google interview questions. A site came up that said, *The 25 most difficult questions you'll be asked on a job interview.* This looked like it was from FOCUS magazine. I couldn't believe my eyes. The exact same questions she asked me were right there! I could have done really well on that interview if I had just spent a little time preparing.

Over the next couple of days, I studied each question and developed a three-part answer to each. I also practiced answering them out loud so that I could get used to hearing myself talk. While answering the question, I would secretly count with my finger which part of the answer I was on. This helped me stay focused and also helped me move on to the next part of my answer smoothly.

I watched myself in the mirror answering the questions. I studied what I did with my hands, how I sat in the chair and even where my eyes looked. I pretended the question was asked and the first thing I did before answering was to look like I was deep in thought. Then I took a nice, deep breath. I realized that one thing I did wrong on the last interview was starve myself of vital oxygen.

I know this because when I was younger my parents put me and my siblings in public speaking contests. My mom and dad watched me practice or perform and that was one of the things they always mentioned. "Caroline, we didn't see you breathe that much and you were talking too fast," my mom would always say. Making a conscious effort to take deep inspirations would help me relax and talk at a reasonable pace.

When I looked at myself in the mirror, I would try to see my teeth as much as possible. I learned this from my first writing workshop. The New York Times bestselling author Andy Andrews was there giving a speech. He spoke for about 30 minutes and he was building up to something. He kept saying that he was going to share the advice that was the most important factor to all of his successes.

We were all thinking his advice was going to be so complicated. But when he said it, I realized some of the best advice is mostly common sense that we forget to make common. "Smile while you talk." That was it. I sat there thinking about it. I had instantly liked him when he first took the stage. Could it be because of his warm smile?

I think that very well could be true. Think about it. When a baby catches your gaze and then gives you a huge smile . . . aren't you instantly in love? On a more scientific level, there's a lot of research being done on mirror neurons inside our brains. Neuroscientist Marco Lacoboni, University of California, contends that that mirror neurons in the human brain help us understand the actions and intentions of other people by assessing things like facial expressions and postures.

It's important that you be genuine in an interview, so even though you practice in a mirror, make sure your smiles are real. In interviewing for the position I wanted, I hoped to give the best service and provide a loving and safe environment. Just thinking about that makes me smile. So, to make sure my smile was not a fake, plastered one, I would envision creating this feeling on the unit that I was applying for.

Another thing I did on the way to the interview was to talk to myself in the car. I imagined I was already in the interview and was already being asked the questions. I think of it like this. Have you ever spent a few hours by yourself and then met up with someone to chat? This can feel weird sometimes, right?

Anything you do, writing, speaking, drawing, there is a period at first where it feels a little awkward. For example, almost every time when I sit down to write, at first I really have to force myself to keep going. But after a few minutes, things flow. It's as though oil enters my mind and the ideas and words just slip out.

Speaking is the same way. If you're going to have an awkward period, why go through it while being interviewed for your dream job, when so much is at stake? Instead, be weird and talk yourself out of that while you're driving to your interview. Don't worry if people see you on the way; they'll just think you're talking to someone on the phone.

The final thing I focused on is the most obvious: What should I wear? My whole goal in mind while making this decision was to choose an outfit that would make people focus on me. The last thing that you want people to say about you was that it looked like you were wearing a $1,000 suit.

Choose an outfit that is more neutral or dark in color and that can make your best features shine in a way that is modest and respectful. If you wear makeup, make sure it, too, is modest, clean and fresh looking. Nothing over the top. Remember, your ultimate goal is to have people remember how you made them feel.

Now, with all of this preparation, how do you think my next interviews went? Needless to say, I got to choose where I wanted to work from multiple offers. But think about it. Had I not pushed myself to apply to a ton of different places, I would never have gotten the rude awakening I really needed.

Ultimately, just remember that interviewing is not something that comes easily to most. Maybe some people are better than others naturally, especially people who are eloquent. But being prepared and having experience makes a huge difference.

Make sure, as I said in Chapter One, that you apply like crazy to every single place that you can. And when the calls start coming in, try to schedule the first interviews at the hospitals you are least interested in. Then you'll be prepared to do a fantastic interview at the places you really want to work!

Caroline Porter Thomas

Chapter 3

Prepare for Your First Nursing JOB!

"There are no secrets to success. It is the result of preparation, hard work, and learning from failure."
– Colin Powell

So you finally made it. You got accepted it into nursing school, you passed nursing school, and you even passed the very, very difficult NCLEX examination. Not only that, you then had to work hard to get an awesome job. But, here you are! You're in uniform and ready to get started on your first job. Now let's prepare so you can be successful at work!

After training several new graduates, I realized that if you step foot on the job knowing a little about what to expect, you'll be better off. I had the pleasure of working with two preceptors. This was an amazing experience because they were each so different, yet they still had the same job and were both excellent nurses.

One of my biggest frustrations when I started was that I wanted to know the RIGHT way to do every task. When I was in nursing school, things were presented in such "matter of fact" ways that I thought that is how it would be in the real world.

One of my preceptors was seriously Ms. Perfect. She did everything very carefully, cautiously and tediously rethinking every task before taking any action. However, she would constantly say, "This is how I do _____." I appreciated that input; however, I really wanted to get down to the bottom of the right way. During my preceptorship, she accepted a job at a different hospital and left.

So my next preceptor was super fun, funny and very scatterbrained. She, too, would say the same thing, "This is how I do _____," as well as every other experienced nurse on the unit. I reluctantly realized that there were multiple ways to start IV's, assess patients, document things and complete almost every other nursing task. You have to choose what works best for you. The only problem is that as a newbie, you don't know all of your options.

When the term "on-the-job training" was mentioned, I didn't realize this meant learning tons of different ways to do one task. Even to this day, when I watch other nurses do something, I'm constantly saying to myself, "That looks better than how I currently do it." And I do it that way from then on.

As a new nurse, you have a lot of work ahead of you, especially for that first six months. It will take you a while to develop a baseline routine that is engrained in you. Once you have that organized, solid routine, you'll be able to handle the variability the days throw at you.

What I have learned about being a nurse is the only thing you can count on is that your mornings will almost always be similar. If you have a well-run morning, the rest of your day usually flows. Afternoons tend to fluctuate depending on: new orders, scheduled medications, patients who need special things (turning, cleaning, dressing changes, blood transfusions) etc. When you first start, your goal is to develop a system where you automatically begin your morning routine. Get your morning things done ASAP because you never know how the rest of your day is going to be.

I like to move as fast as possible in the mornings. I mean physically, mentally, everything. However, there is one thing I say to myself over and over, "I first have to be safe.'' I've learned to automatically get my patients' morning medications from the med room and while walking to my patients' rooms, actually look at each medication and see if it is appropriate. I have Lopressor for my patient, so what was her blood pressure and heart rate? Next medication is potassium, so what was his level this morning?

Computer charting makes all of these questions usually very easy to answer. However, if you still use paper, just make an effort to stop at the main chart to look at information that will help you be safe. I would venture to say that 70% of your work is done in the morning, which is why I place so much focus on that part of your day.

Here is my baseline morning routine:
1st get my assignment.
2nd check my patients' labs.
3rd Get report in the room and greet my patient
4th Either get or check my patients' morning vital signs.
5th Pull my first patients' medications (if everyone is ok, I usually just go with the earliest medication scheduled).
6th while giving meds, I do a quick head to toe assessment and document it immediately.
7th See all patients, give their medications, assess & document.

This routine, of course, depends on the acuity of my patients, how many medications they have and what else is going on. These seven steps alone can take me anywhere from 1 ½ hours to 3 hours. At this point, I usually have a lot of new orders to follow up on (if you work night shift, you usually will not have as many new orders). What is good is that you do the same things over and over.

To help me keep tabs on my progress, I have a sticky note with all of my patient's rooms on it. I check by each name as I finish the baseline routine. I do not rely on the computer system to help me keep track, because every now and again it doesn't work right; When you start computer documentation, you'll understand. So just to make sure, I still rely heavily on my sticky notes.

New graduates usually begin by taking care of one to two patients. Use this time to get used to the baseline routine. Follow the above steps so they become habit. During the individual assessments, get a baseline orientation and use your stethoscope to check their chests. After that, my stethoscope is on their stomach, accompanied by the question "When was your last BM and are you having difficulty urinating?"

After that, without even thinking, my hands check their pulses and seeing if they are edematous. Once my hands are on their ankles to check for edema, I'm triggered to remember exactly why this patient is in the room. Did they just have surgery, were they having chest pain, are they here for pneumonia? Once I remember that, I finish with my skin assessment where I examine any abnormalities my patient may have.

Once I have finished my assessment, I document it right there in the room. This may be difficult as a new graduate, but you want to get to the point where documenting your main assessment takes less than 5 minutes. Also at that point, you can usually document your Morris falls score because you're in the room and you can ask them if they have fallen. The

Braden score will just take you a second too. If you're not familiar with them, the Morris Falls score assesses your patient's risk for falling and the Braden tool assesses your patient's risk for developing a pressure ulcer.

And since you're going to be giving the morning medications, document your education right there too. What I usually do is go through the medications one by one and ask them if they are not familiar with any of them. If they say yes then I go over that medication, explaining the therapeutic benefits as well as some of the most common side effects. This usually just takes a minute and offers some education you can document.

When you start and have few patients, make sure you look up every medication that you're not familiar with, which may be every medication. What I like to do is go to the recommended resource on the computer screen and read the information. Then I also like to ask an experienced nurse about the medication. I usually ask them the same questions just to make sure I read the information correctly: What is this medication for, is there anything that I need to do before giving it and is there anything I need to look for after administration.

What you will find is that each unit gives many of the same medications over and over. In the beginning, you may look up 20 to 30 different medications. However, once these medications become familiar, you'll have fewer and fewer medications to look up. But make sure it's a habit to look up every medication you don't know.

Make it a habit by making it easy. It's habit to click on the recommended resource link on the computer screen for me. This way I read really quickly. If I still don't understand, which does happen, I call pharmacy and speak to a pharmacist and then also to speak with an experienced nurse. Making these actions habits in your routine helps you not stress over new medications.

After being a nurse for five years, I still regularly look up medications. Every now and then there are days that I give only familiar medications. However, usually about once or twice a shift, I come across a medication name that I'm not familiar with and have to rely on my habits.

As a new graduate when you have one to four patients, you're going to have a lot of free time. This is expected. I've seen new graduates use this time very ineffectively and also very wisely. It's not effective if you're sitting down talking about non-work related subjects.

There is a time and place when you can do this, but make every attempt not to let this happen while you're on orientation. I know that I have written down the steps like they are no brainers, but don't underestimate the complexity of the job. It will take you at least six months to feel somewhat comfortable… it actually took me eight months. The harder you push yourself now, the easier it will be later. The opposite is also true.

Here are a few things you can do make sure you utilize your preceptorship and training at the highest level. Write this list down and look at it frequently.

1. Stick close to your preceptor and ask tons of questions.
2. Ask other nurses if they have anything good for a new graduate to see.
3. Run to every single emergency.
4. Help everyone around you to build your team.

Let's talk about each step. The first is to stick close to your preceptor and ask tons of questions. Remember, you're taking a little bit of the workload off of them. Their main job is to be your resource. Directors do put a lot of time and thought into who they place you with… however, if you have a preceptor who makes you feel bad when you ask questions or follow her or him around, you may want to talk with someone about it. First, of course, explain to your preceptor that being new, you're very nervous and just want to be a good and safe nurse. Usually if you talk a little bit about what is bothering you, your preceptor may remember what it was like when he or she started and be more sympathetic.

The next step is to ask other nurses to let you know if they have a good learning experience for a new graduate. There are so many different nursing tasks to learn that there is no way you and your preceptor can be assigned to everything, so make sure you start your morning by talking to all of the nurses and letting them know you're eager to learn.

The third is to run to every emergency. When you see a patient in distress for the first time, you may not recognize what this looks like. I know it sounds like common sense but for me it was not. Listen for these words: Medical Response Team (MRT), or STAT team or Rapid Response, whatever your hospital calls it. This is the code called when a nurse thinks the patient may be declining, but it's not as severe as a Code Blue. And, of course, if you also hear a Code Blue, go to that as well.

Under these emergent situations you'll see the role of the primary nurse. That nurse may be the only person in the room who knows the patient. Basically what happens is once the emergency is called, the charge nurse on the unit comes to help out and maybe one or two co-workers. Then you usually have the physician on call, a few critical care nurses and the nursing supervisor.

The first question that is going to be asked of the primary nurse is "What is going on?" That nurse really needs to give the SBAR response, which is Situation, Background, Assessment and Recommendation. This is invaluable experience because one day you will be that primary nurse. So experience as many of these as possible.

The last step is to help absolutely everyone around you. This includes but is not limited to your nursing assistant, your preceptor, other nurses and even the charge nurse. Verbally tell everyone that you are here if they need any assistance with anything. You won't believe how grateful people will be. And believe me, down the road you will also need their assistance, so use this time to gain rapport with every person on the unit.

Caroline Porter Thomas

Chapter 4

What to Bring With You

"By failing to prepare, you are preparing to fail."
Benjamin Franklin

If I do something on a daily basis, I figure out a way to make it a habit. Whenever a new task is added or I start to see a new medication more often that requires something specific, I find a way to make administration easier. For example, let's just say our hospital started ordering Dilaudid IV 2 mg in a glass vial. I will start carrying with me filtered needles so that I'm not running up and down the unit looking for a filtered needle while my patient suffers in pain.

I'm very methodical about how and where I place things in my pockets. Because my goal every day is to move faster and faster on the unit, this involves knowing where everything is that I need to get my job done. I take what I do very seriously. I'm grateful every single time that I have the opportunity to care for an individual. I am so grateful for the hospital and the administrators who run the organization that gives me a place to do this awesome job. You should feel the same; I know you worked hard for this, but it is still a privilege. With that said, let me tell you how I prepare to do an outstanding job.

I'm going to first list the supplies that I keep in my pocket on a regular basis:

Caroline Porter Thomas

Left Shirt Pocket
1. Alcohol swabs
2. Sticky notepad
3. Flushes
4. Wrapped 18 gauge blunt needles   2 or 3
5. Filtered needles 2 or 3
6. Empty 3 ml syringe 1 or 2
7. Telemetry leads 1 or 2
8. On the outside I have a banana hair clip

Right Shirt Pocket
1. Scissors
2. Highlighter
3. Black dry erase marker
4. Red dry erase marker
5. Black Sharpie
6. Mechanical multicolor pen
7. 2 mechanical pencils
8. One pink (or turquoise) uni-ball pen
9. 2 black mechanical pens
10. Transparent tape
11. Pen light
12. Telemetry calipers

In my pants pockets
1. Pulse oximeter (right pocket)
2. Temporal thermometer (left pocket)

In my bag
1. Pill crusher
2. Another pair of medical scissors

Each item is important to my work. I usually work as a Telemetry/Cardiac nurse. I say "usually" because I am also a float nurse, which means I can go to multiple units. I have been floating for almost three years now, so I am trained for a number of different specialties. I am giving you my base list; however, keep in mind that for your specialty, this equipment list may vary quite a bit. The main goal is to have your frequently used items available so you can do your job in a timely manner.

The first item on the list is alcohol swabs. I have no idea how many I use on a daily basis, but I start out with about 1-inch thick handful of the double packets and usually around 2 p.m. have to reload. I also know that most of the time alcohol swabs are commonly found items on the unit. Well, I have had so many days where there isn't one to be found, so no way am I starting my day like that. This is seriously one of the biggest infection control measures (after hand washing, of course), so just have some on you.

A sticky notepad is the next item on the list. I am very task oriented and like to check things off as I go along. I have also noted that we can get extremely busy on the job and it's easy to overlook minor things. For example, you have a patient whose blood pressure is at a level you never thought imaginable. So you're calling the doctor, giving medications, assessing your patient. Then another patient asks you for water.

What I have learned about being a nurse and making your patients happy is that it's the little things that matter most. You can get your patient's blood pressure down, you can notify the doctor about their low potassium and replace it, you can notice a jump in their white blood cell count that the doctor missed and get an order for an infection control doctor to be on the case. But, make getting water for your patients a priority and they will love you forever. Most likely they will never know 90% of what you do for them. But if you bring them something basic that they asked for, they remember that.

How do I remember how to do everything? If I relied on myself, I would be completely lost. At any given moment (especially in the morning), I could have between 10 to 20 really important things on my mind. If possible, I just do the task right then and there, and try to walk as fast as possible. If not, I use my sticky notes immediately and plaster it on my notebook. What gets placed on that notebook, via sticky notes, will get done.

I also make it a point to keep track of my morning progress with the sticky notes as I mentioned in the previous chapter. Again, I write down my room numbers and check them off as I finish their morning medications and assessments. Once everyone has a check, all of my morning medications and assessments are finished. That sticky note gets placed in the trash… and man does that feel good.

Saline flushes are the next item on the list. I carry two to three with me just in case I forgot one, or if I need to check an IV to make sure it's still working or patent. These are one of the biggest items you carry so you won't be able to carry everything you need all the time. What I do is gather all of my patient's medications and, if they have an IV medication, I grab the flushes I need for that time.

The 18-gauge needles to draw up medications you will probably use tons of times during the day. I like to use the same method as the flushed and just carry a few with me just in case. But when I'm gathering my patient's medications, I also grab the needles for that specific trip.

The filtered needles may be another story. You will most likely not use these all the time. However, when you need them sometimes they are nowhere to be found. I still remember the day I ran around for 20 minutes looking for one. I had a patient with end-stage pancreatic cancer and she asked me for her pain medicine. The doctor had ordered Dilaudid 2 mg IV every 3 hours.

The time was appropriate and she asked for it. No problem, I told her. I grabbed the medication immediately and it was in the glass vial. So I went to the supply room for a filtered needle, and here wasn't one to be found. I asked other nurses to also look just in case I missed them. I didn't. I went to three other units in the hospital before I finally found one.

By the time I got to my patient's room, she was crying so loud and was in so much pain that I felt terrible. Her whole family was also in the room and they were crying too. It was heartbreaking to listen to her suffer and I also teared up. I composed myself enough to efficiently give her the medication as soon as safely possible.

This was the first time I saw someone in such uncontrollable pain. Had I just had a filtered needle around, I could have given the medication just minutes after she asked. I said to myself that day, how can I make sure this never happens to anyone else? And the answer was to keep a filtered needle close.

The empty 3-ml syringes are just in case I have a medication that you're not supposed to dilute with saline. I only carry one or two of these with me. This really is not high on the priority list.

As a cardiac monitoring nurse, I seriously must have leads with me. Leads are the little stickers you place on your patient's chest that connect to a portable or in the room heart monitor. This gives us a view of what is going on with the patient's heart at any given time. These are super small stickers and it's really easy to have three to four of these. Theoretically if the doctor has ordered for your patient to be on continuous cardiac monitoring, then your patient should not ever be off the monitor.

However, these little stickies easily come loose with a little body oil, sweat, hair or movement. If your patient happens to have or do all four above, then they can be nearly impossible to keep on. Keeping a few of these on you is a good idea just in case you need to make a quick stop to replace it so there is little interruption of monitoring data.

For the ladies (maybe gents as well) who like to wear their long hair down at times, a banana clip is a great item. I love having my hair down for most of the day. However, there are definitely times when it's not appropriate or it gets in the way. Having a banana clip on my pocket helps me place my hair up in seconds. And it looks great too!

So let's move to the right shirt pocket. The very first item I have listed is scissors. These are medical scissors; however, I use these only for medications. What I learned from being a nurse is that actually getting your medications can sometimes be challenging. Especially Colace! Why is that? By now, you may have seen enough to know what I'm talking about. But each pill is separated and placed on a sheet with other pills. Just tearing these apart can literally be painful. So in order to make it easier, I just cut with my scissors instead of trying to pull them apart anymore. As I said, though, I use these for medication and clean things only. In my bag I have another pair if I need to do anything else.

My list contains a lot of writing utensils. I use every one of those items a lot. The highlighter for things I want to remember. The black and red dry erase markers are to keep the patients' blackboards updated. The black sharpie is just in case I need to label anything. The multi-colored pen is also to highlight. The pencils I use especially when I'm getting report, just in case I hear something wrong.

The transparent tape is something you'll want with you in order to secure a few things; IV's are the main things I find myself reinforcing often. When you lose one of those because it wasn't secure, it's a lot of work to replace. So play it safe and keep a small roll with you.

The pen light is one of those items that you want to keep with you just in case of an emergency. If you notice a patient declining, the worst-case scenario is you see changes in their pupils. To make sure your patient's pupils are equal and reactive to light, keep a pen light close.

In my pants pockets, I have two very important items that I recommend you buy. The first is a pulse oximeter, which measures the amount of oxygen that your body is absorbing. The second is a temporal thermometer.

Caroline Porter Thomas

I carry the pulse oximeter because good supplies are sometimes hard to find in the hospital setting. However, you want to give your patient the best care possible, right?

Remember you passed the NCLEX examination, which basically says that you are a safe practitioner. Part of being safe is knowing that your patient's vital signs are within normal or acceptable limits according to their health. One day, I had a patient who told me he was having difficulty breathing. I ran up and down the hallways looking for the vital sign machine so I could check my patient. It seemed like it took 20 minutes, but probably only took one minute.

Think about it, though. If someone tells you they're having difficulty breathing, isn't one minute too long? As I walked up and down the halls, I asked the same question to myself. "How can I make sure this never happens again?" I noticed the respiratory therapists all had small pulse oximeters. I also had a patient in the past with bad pulmonary sarcoidosis who wore a pulse oximeter to make sure he breathed enough when needed.

So I thought how hard could it be for me to get my own? It was even easier than I thought. For just about $60, I got one from my local CVS. The peace of mind it gives me is absolutely priceless. At least I know if my patient is ok or not. I cannot tell you how many times I have a patient who tells me they can't breathe. I check them and they are 99% oxygen saturation on room air. I just tell them that, they relax and they're fine.

Of course, the opposite is also true. If your patient doesn't look too hot, just check their saturation level. You can tell a lot by that number; if it is 92 or below, you need to do something about that. Place your patient on 2L, listen to their lungs, call a respiratory therapist and the doctor. It's just so freeing, though, that you can know right away instead of running up and down the halls, looking for equipment.

In my left pants pocket I carry a temporal thermometer. The reason for this is very similar to the rationale behind the pulse oximeter. Basically, one day I really needed to check my patient's temperature and couldn't find one vital sign machine. So I made sure I'm always able to know my patient's temperature. Since it is temporal, I just have to scan my patient's forehead and then clean it with the sterilizing wipes.

In my bag, I have two items that I don't use every day. The first is a pill crusher, which is used for obvious reasons. The other one is another pair of medical scissors. These are the scissors I use for any "dirty work." The main thing I use them for is dressing changes. I do try everything my power not to use them; first of all, I check everywhere to see if there is already a pair in the patient's room, or if there is a pair in the supply room. If not, though, I just have to use my own and clean them like crazy when I'm done.

So those are the items I carry with me to make my challenging job a little more doable. I hope this list helps you. Just make sure you take note anytime you are wasting precious time walking up and down the hallways for something you could already have with you.

Caroline Porter Thomas

Chapter 5

What to Wear on the Job

Dress to impress and never let them see your frown. Cause there are people who would kill to see you down.

- Unknown Author

In today's hospital climate, there is little room for creativity as far as scrubs go. The majority of hospitals are mandating uniforms. Even if your hospital doesn't do so, this chapter will be beneficial for you. What I have realized is that you still have flexibility regarding certain parts of your appearance.

When I first became a nurse five years ago, I definitely dressed differently than I do today. My style has morphed into a different theme. I say *theme* very purposefully. When I am preparing myself for the day, I have an overlying theme that I want to represent to my boss, my colleagues and for my own satisfaction. My focus when I first started was that I wanted to look very attractive, intelligent and stand out.

Since I wanted to stand out, I wore bright earrings and a little more makeup than necessary. Since my intent was to look attractive, I always had my hair looking its best. I remember nurses always asking me what time I woke up to get ready. It really didn't take that long since I had a pretty good routine down.

I stood out for sure. There were very few nurses that put any effort at all into themselves. Many of them told me that they were just planning on doing dirty work all day, so what was the point in looking good. They would show up without a drop of makeup on, their hair in a pony tail and bags under their eyes.

My parents always put a lot of emphasis on our appearance. Not for my siblings and me to be super attractive, but for us to look as though we care about how the world perceives us. They said that if you look your best, you will do your best. This was the mantra I have carried with me my entire life. I know that I wear scrubs. But there are not scrubs on my face (although I know surgical nurses or nurses in other specialties may have to wear masks).

However, since I was young and wanted to see if it was the truth about looking your best, I decided to do an experiment. For 1 month, I decided to sleep in an extra 30 minutes, wake up and not put any effort into my appearance, besides the minor things like wearing a wrinkle-free uniform. I thought maybe they were right, maybe the extra 30 minutes of sleep would be better than putting that 30 minutes into myself.

I did it. I woke up, threw my hair in a pony tail and put my scrubs on. I went to work without putting any effort into my appearance. I told myself that my main focus was my patients and it didn't matter how I looked. I didn't vary my routine any; I wanted to give myself a very real vision of what these habits would feel like. I began to hate my job.

When I had a patient who would complain about the care they were given., I would say to myself, "Nurses sacrifice themselves for you." I was less patient and also less in tune with myself. I realized that during the 30 minutes that I was putting on makeup and doing my hair, I was also talking to myself and seeing how I wanted my day to go.

So about two weeks into my experiment, I decided that it was not how I looked but the energy I put into myself in the morning that made the difference. So, what if I woke up the same 30 minutes early and meditated? This was very helpful. I would spend that time visualizing how grateful I was for all of my patients, my co-workers and my bosses. I still didn't put any effort into my appearance and did the same pony tail and no makeup. It still was not the same. I was not as in love with my job as before.

Those 30 days on the job were so long. I felt like I didn't matter, that I was unattractive and put my patients above myself. Many people think that sacrificing yourself is an honorable thing to do. I do not think this is a good long-term habit. I've learned that if you sacrifice yourself for someone else, you judge their every behavior. You think about the energy and effort that your sacrifice cost and, if they don't respond appropriately, you may begin to resent them.

When you're on an airplane, they always instruct you to place your own oxygen first. They understand that if you do not take care of yourself first, you can't help anyone else. What I was doing in the morning by putting my makeup on and doing my hair was giving myself love, filling myself up. Then I was able to fill other people up.

So now when I put the energy and effort into myself, for the most part, I still want to look attractive and intelligent. But now that I'm older, I also realize on this job how important it is to come across as caring, compassionate and put together. Those are the thoughts that are going through my mind as I prepare for my day. By the time I get to my work, I'm so filled up with all of this that I am able to give abundantly. The bottom line is to look at every detail of your appearance and look your absolute best, so you will do your best.

Next, I want to talk about the actual uniform. When hospitals mandate this, it's usually only the color and sometimes brand that matter. For example, one hospital asked us to wear Cherokee Royal Blue. So they mandated a brand and a color; however, within the brand and color there were a lot of options. There are so many different types of pants and tops it is really unbelievable.

Here is my advice to you. I always buy the same pants and tops. The reason for this is simple. When one day your shirt has five pockets and the next day two, or your pants you wore yesterday had a side leg pocket, but today's pants don't, it is inconsistent. Little things like these can irritate you when you're really busy.

Here is how I buy my scrubs. Whether I am online or at the store, I pick the one shirt I like and the one pair of pants I like, and then buy three of each. I also always buy scrub jackets to match, so three of these as well. This way I'm set for the entire week and I only have to do laundry once.

Now that all of your scrub tops and bottoms are the same, decide where you want to place your items. Obviously, this may take a little while because you are new, but as you go along your day, make sure you think about this. As I listed the items I carry with me in the previous chapter, did you notice how I categorized them by pocket?

When I need an alcohol swab, I know where to go. If I do not have an alcohol swab right there, I don't have one! No need to search all of my pockets; just go get more. Also, here is another example on why to organize your pockets. When your patients ask you for something for pain, you go get the medication from the machine. While you are walking back, your co-worker asks you to do a little favor and help turn her patient. Since you are so nice, you do it.

But what about the narcotic you had in your hand? So I always place any narcotics in the same place, no matter what. Believe me, these ideas sound simple when you are just reading this, but things can get really busy and if you learn to automate things now, it will make your job easier later.

Caroline Porter Thomas

Chapter 6

How to Read Doctor's Notes

"Learn avidly. Question repeatedly what you have learned. Analyze it carefully. Then put what you have learned into practice intelligently." – Edward Cocker

One of the main nursing roles is to be the mediator between doctors and patients. Many times when your patient was visited by their doctor and then, after the doctor leaves, your patient asks you what the plan is. I've had many patients say that they didn't want to ask their doctor a question because they didn't want to look stupid. But they feel safe asking me the questions. Also, many times they can repeat verbatim what the doctor's plan is for them; however, they have no idea what it all means.

That's why we are here. To clarify any questions our patients have concerning their care; it is one of our main roles. The only problem is that rarely are we with the doctors and patients during their visits, and we hardly ever are visited by the doctor directly after the visit. So how do we know what their plan is?

Thankfully nowadays with computer charting, most doctors type up their notes. There are a few old-school doctors who are still fighting the computer documentation tooth and nail, but I have a feeling they soon will lose this fight. This allows a doctor to write his progress note, and once the note is saved we can see it immediately. Many computer charting systems will also alert you once a progress note is made by any physician on the case.

This allows you to stay up to date with your patient's care. Believe me, these notes come in handy. There will be many times when you are extremely busy and say that you'll notify a doctor once they get to the unit. Somehow, though, you missed them, and they managed to round on the entire unit and you were so busy that you didn't see them. There have been countless times when I've had situations that weren't life threatening or didn't require a doctor's attention immediately, but that they would eventually need to know.

For example, let's say that your patient's WBC's are higher today than yesterday despite the antibiotics they are on. Or let's say that your patient's potassium is just slightly low and your patient could use a replacement, but this particular doctor only likes to be awakened up during the night if something is really life threatening. Or do they still know your patient is NPO?

If you work at a teaching facility, which I have, the doctor situation is absolutely wonderful. With just the dial of a number, you can notify a doctor on your patient's case and take the order, if needed, immediately. Sometimes however if you work at hospitals that don't participate in this, you'll have to notify the attending physician. It may be much harder to get a call back.

Understanding what type of facility you work at will help you plan your patient's care. But let's just say you're working at a hospital that isn't a teaching facility. And, just to make it interesting, every nurse on the unit knows that this doctor only wants to be notified if someone is dying. Although you need to practice safe nursing and do whatever it takes to take care of your patient, there are some things you can do before you get on the phone and get yelled at.

Whenever you are new to a unit, which of course you are now as a recent graduate, ask the seasoned nurses around you about the physician. Sometimes doctors will have what are called "Standing Orders" for simple medications such as Tylenol or Milk of Magnesia. This means that you can write the order for the medication without contacting the physician.

Also, some doctors don't respond to your call unless you page them or contact them in a certain way. Unfortunately, the main channel to get this information is through the nurses on the unit. That's why I always ask beforehand. I find myself asking these questions all the time because I float to different hospitals and different units. I work for a staffing agency that does supplemental staffing for many hospitals in the S. Florida region.

Here is an example of something that has happened to me numerous times. Once my morning vital signs were taken, I noticed that my patient's blood pressure was super elevated. He had a history of hypertension so fortunately morning blood pressure medications were ordered. I gave his medications immediately and then rechecked in 1 hour. Still high.

I looked through his medication list and noticed he has a PRN blood pressure medication. I gave that and then rechecked the blood pressure in 1 hour. Still very high. At this point, I need to get a hold of the physician. I paged the doctor and while I waited, I tried to determine if there was anything else I could do. I noticed the patient was on IVF; he was here for renal failure, too, and could benefit from the hydration; however, now it seemed as though the patient wasn't able to handle the extra hydration.

I also noticed my patient was super nervous, probably from me checking his blood pressure so much. I sat down and talked with him and reminded him to take nice slow deep breaths. I turned Jerry Springer off and made sure he didn't have any pain, which can elevate blood pressure.

I then noticed it had been 15 minutes and the doctor hadn't called me back. I took my patient's blood pressure again to have an accurate reading for the doctor, and I paged him again. Each time I page a physician, I prepare a sticky note so I'm able to notify him or her of the situation in an organized fashion. We'll discuss this in depth in the next chapter. However, for now, I just want to note that it's very important to keep track of the time you last paged the doctor so you can re-page him or her as soon as appropriate (unless it's critical, of course).

By the 3rd time I paged this particular physician, with no response back, I went to the charge nurse and asked if there was a better way to get in touch of this physician. She answered, "Oh, Dr. Smith only likes to be called on his cell. He never answers his pages." Well, wouldn't that have been great to know 45 minutes ago? I called the cell phone and would you believe that Dr. Smith answered immediately?

Once you work on a unit for a few months, you start to learn about all of the physicians and how they operate. This information is helpful and important so that you can care for your patients appropriately. Until you know the information yourself, make sure you ask the surrounding nurses their previous experiences with the doctors. I mention this because much of the information can be found in the doctor's notes; before you call the physician, you can see if they mentioned whether the patient has uncontrolled blood pressure.

While reading the notes, you'll notice that most of them use the same format. I've worked in three different states at probably more than 20 different hospitals and have noticed the same overall platform. It goes in this order: Subjective assessment, Objective assessment, Diagnosis and Plan. The words may not always be the same, but most doctors follow approximately the same outline.

Let's go over this: The subjective assessment is what the patient states to the physician. The physician asks the patient how they are feeling today. The patients may say they are still in pain, or still nauseous or that they are feeling much better than before. The physician may ask them how they slept. The admitting diagnosis will be a huge factor in determining the questions that they will ask to.

They may mention if the patient is complying with the care plan the doctor is ordering; they may also ask if the patient needs to take additional medications such as for pain or anxiety. At this point, they may also ask us, the nurses in charge of care, if the patient had any complaints or if there were any issues overnight. If this was about the patient above, we would mention the patient's blood pressure and tell all of the measures we took to control it.

Caroline Porter Thomas

The next section of the note is the objective information, like vital signs, lab values, radiology reports and the doctor's findings on his/her assessment. They usually just copy and paste all of the patient's vital signs and lab values. Most of them also copy and paste the lab values, too, and many of them, depending on their specialty, also paste the radiology findings. If you want to know if your doctor is aware of your patient's high blood pressure, see if they noted it here.

They also list their assessment of all systems: EENT (Eyes, Ears, Nose, Throat) , cardiovascular, respiratory, gastrointestinal, genitourinary, musculoskeletal, integumentary, neurological, psychiatric, endocrine, hematologic/lymphatic and allergic/immunologic. Many times doctors will do what nurses do and chart by exception. So if they don't mention anything under the respiratory system but they put a note under the cardiovascular system, in theory the respiratory system of your patient should be fine.

Also depending on the acuity of the patient, doctors in general will do a much more in-depth assessment on their sicker patients. If you work on a Med-Surg unit, your notes may be brief with little information listed under your review of systems. And if you work on an Intensive Care Unit, you may have very long notes with comments and plans under every single system. Of course, because you care for fewer patients on the ICU unit, you will have time to read these detailed notes... hopefully.

So after all of the subjective and objective data, the doctor should have arrived at a diagnosis and plan. The diagnosis may or may not be the same as the admitting diagnosis. Sometimes patients are admitted under a certain diagnosis and then that is ruled out, and physicians may change the diagnosis. The plan should follow and that is one of the most helpful pieces in the entire note for you.

Being the mediator between patient and physician, you can use these notes to help you stay updated with your patient's care. I cannot tell you how many times I get a call from the secretary and she says. "Caroline, Ms. Jennings's husband is at the desk and he wants an update. He is waiting in the patient's room for you." My first response is, Who is Jennings? And then I remember, oh yes, she is the only patient who has been super quiet and stable today.

Just taking 2 minutes to read the doctor's notes, I can go into Mrs. Jennings's room and update them on their care. It's that easy. Many times all the information I need is located in the last paragraph under the "Plan" section, and that is usually all the patient and family want to know. Of course, it's good to open the computer while you are in the room if you need to just in case they have more in-depth questions.

Caroline Porter Thomas

Chapter 7

How to Approach Doctors

"If there is any great secret of success in life, it lies in the ability to put yourself in the other person's place and to see things from his point of view – as well as your own. "

Henry Ford

When you start out as a nurse, you'll see other nurses approach doctors in different ways. Some nurses are just able to call a doctor after memorizing everything they needed to ask, and the conversation goes smoothly. These are usually nurses with a lot of experience, both in nursing and in that particular hospital, working with that specific doctor. You will also see the opposite, super scatterbrained nurses who will page the doctor and then scramble through their notes when they get a call back.

The nurse-doctor relationship is all about how you communicate. You may see nurses getting upset with physicians; physicians getting upset with nurses. It's funny because sometimes I will be sitting right there, listening to the whole conversation. I'll hear the nurse speak to the doctor and nine times out of 10, if she's unhappy with the call, I believe the way she handled the conversation had a lot to do with it.

Your organization, voice tone, pitch and speed at which you converse have more to do with the response you get back than anything else. Remember, you are a busy person. If someone had to call you for something, wouldn't it be great if they were pleasant, organized and to the point?

I agree that every now and then you may have a doctor, Physicians Assistant or Nurse Practitioner call you back who is blatantly rude. However, I guarantee if you have your information straight, then this will happen one out of every 1,000 calls you receive back. Also, if you remain calm no matter how they treat you, they will treat you differently next time.

The key here is to never judge anyone by the way they interact with you on the phone or in person. First of all, you have no idea what that person is going through. The physician's job is very difficult. They see many, many patients, have to deal with demanding family members, often must tell patients bad news and work very long hours. What if you were to call a physician right after he told a patient that he had end-stage cancer, and the patient's family was screaming at him saying that it was his fault for not catching it earlier. The bottom line is that you need to be respectful of their time, just as you would like it if people did the same for you.

As a new nurse, I made several mistakes that led me to the method that I now use. I hope you use this method so you can learn from my mistakes. Depending on where you work and how it is appropriate to communicate with physicians, i.e. beeper, phone etc., adjustments must be made accordingly. For example, if you can call the physician directly, more pre-planning needs to be done, and if you happen to page the doctor you usually have a few minutes (sometimes much longer) before they call you back.

When you are paging a doctor about a situation, ask yourself a series of questions before you speak to them. What I do is take out a sticky note, and write the patient's name and room number at the top. Then write the physician's name and number (just in case I have to page them again), followed by notations of the exact time, every time, I page them. I then write down the reason for the page, for example, elevated Blood Pressure (BP) that did not get better after the morning medications were given.

I write down the patient's BP and also the patient's heart rate (HR) because there are many medications that help lower the BP, but also affect the HR. I then ask myself, what other information would the doctor need to know. Assume the doctor doesn't know anything about your patient because many times this is the case. So I then write down the admitting diagnosis, any medications given that could have affected the BP or HR. Is my patient on IV fluids? Do they have a history of hypertension?

Since I am paging the physician anyway, I then ask myself if there's anything else I may need to communicate with the physician about later. I take a quick glance at my patient's labs, vital sign trend and then I finally go to my patient and ask them a few questions. Here is what I would say: ''Mrs. Smith, I noticed that your blood pressure is a little higher today than it was the last few days. Is there anything bothering you today, or are you in pain? Also, I want your doctor to know so I'm going to contact him/her. While I'm on the phone with them, is there anything else you need?''

Going into my patient's room and talking to them saves me many pages in the future. I cannot tell you how many times I've had patients tell me things like, "Oh yes, I was going to have you contact the doctor later because I wanted something for my dry eyes, or sore throat…" There are usually a lot of little things that would make your patient's stay more comfortable, but you don't necessarily want to page your doctor 10 times a day for. This is your chance; you have to contact them anyway so get the orders for the little things.

So how do you know what questions to ask? Well, experience does help, there is no doubt about that. While you're on orientation, take advantage of your nursing preceptor. Or if you're finished with orientation and you're paging a physician you've never contacted before, ask an experienced nurse if there is any more information that they know of that the doctor may need.

Never underestimate the helpfulness of other people's experiences. Listening to the mistakes other people have made can prove to be invaluable in your learning process. This is why in these next few paragraphs I will include a list of mistakes I've personally made in my five years as a nurse, as well as the lessons I have learned from them.

One time I paged the doctor about my patient's elevated BP like the story above. This time, however, that was all we discussed. He quickly gave me an order for Atenolol 25mg to be given now, and then daily. So I took the order and scanned it to pharmacy. When I was about to give the medication, I repeated my patient's BP check. It was still elevated. However, I forgot to tell the doctor that this patient was Brady on the monitor and his resting HR was 51. So I had to page the doctor again and get an order for a medication that would not slow down the heart rate more, as well as to cancel the previous order.

I wish I could tell you that this has only happened once in my entire career as a nurse. We get so busy, have to page multiple physicians, have so many other people calling us all the time that minor details like this can easily be overlooked. This was an easy thing to fix, especially since the medication was not given. However, it takes a lot of time to page and then re-page a physician. So remember to look at all of your patient's vital signs (VS) before you page the doctor.

The next scenario that I will give is this. One day my patient asked me to call her doctor for something for her heartburn. No problem, I said. I then asked her a few questions. When did it start, how long have you had it, is this the first time you've ever had this. She said it started after lunch, and it has persisted for about two hours now. She said she's had this in the past and it wasn't new. I paged the physician and told him all of this information. The first question he asked was, "Does she take something at home?" Oh yeah, of course. I had to stop what I was doing and run back into the patient's room to find out.

"Yes," she said. "At home, I take Prilosec 40 mg every morning." You would think that this would have been the first piece of information she would have told me. However, really, it should have been the first question I asked. So now I have learned that whenever a patient asks me to call a doctor for a medication for antacid or any other medication, the first question I ask is, "Do you take anything at home?"

Just to give you a little heads up, our geriatric population is often very set on having bowel movements every day, which is good. However, when they're in the hospital many times, they're off their normal routine and things do not move to their approval. So when they ask you to call their doctor for something to help them get going, remember to ask, "Do you take anything at home that works for you?" You would be surprised the number of people who have something they take on a regular basis. And if you know that works for them, see if their doctor will give you an order for it.

Now I'll tell you about my patient who was having pain in her left ankle. She said that from walking around the halls all day she is super sore and would like something for pain. I asked her if this was a new experience for her and she told me that wasn't. I asked how long she has had it, to describe the pain and if she takes anything at home for it. She told me she's had the pain the entire three days she has been here, but now it's getting worse. She described it as a soreness when she walks on that ankle, and she also told me her doctor told her to just take over–the-counter ibuprofen.

I paged her doctor and heard back from her after three pages, which I did over the course of about an hour. Once she called me back, I spoke with the doctor and the first question she had for me was what dose and how often does the patient take ibuprofen. So, of course, I had to again stop what I was doing and go ask the patient that information.

This next story about one of my experiences shows how we can become super focused on what we think is wrong and forget to ask ourselves the obvious questions. One day my nursing assistant ran up to me and said, "Your patient in 312 A, her blood pressure is really low 85/49 and she is profusely sweating." I ran in the room to assess my patient. She was indeed sweating; I rechecked her pressure and it was roughly the same. This particular patient was non-verbal so I wasn't able to learn subjective information.

I looked at the patient's trends in blood pressures and she normally ran in the 130s over 60s. So this was indeed low for her. Once I reached the physician on the phone, the first question she asked was,"What is the patient's blood glucose (BG)?" Of course that should have been one of my first thoughts; I ran and grabbed the glucometer and her BG was 55. We gave her some dextrose, adjusted her IV fluids and she was fine from that point on.

Another scenario I want to share with you is one that happens all of the time. You'll have a patient who wants you to call the doctor to see if their IV fluids could be stopped. They will say things like I feel much better now, I just want to walk around without having to drag this machine, the tubing is getting caught on everything, etc. I would check things like their labs and see if they were dehydrated when they came in by evidence of their BUN & creatinine. I would also look at their admitting diagnosis; sometimes if they come in for vomiting, doctors will order it.

Once I get a hold of the doctor, nine times out of 10 they ask me if the patient is tolerating liquids and food. I rarely if ever make that mistake anymore, but this is just to give you an example.

Anther request you'll get is for nicotine patches. Did you know there are different doses of the patch depending on how much you smoke? Well, there are, so the first question you need to ask when your patient ask for a patch is, "How much do you smoke on a regular basis?" They will say things like one pack per day or five cigarettes per day. This will give the doctor the information they need to order the correct dose to alleviate cravings.

Another mistake I've made multiple times when my patient wants me to call the doctor to let him know that they can't urinate. I page the doctor and her first question is, "Have you performed a bladder scan?" This, by the way, is an amazing piece of equipment. It is similar to the ultrasound that pregnant women get to see their baby, only the equipment is much smaller. You hold the small handheld piece over the bladder and it tells you how much fluid there is.

This is a nursing intervention that you do not need a doctor's order for. Imagine how much easier it would be for you to be able to tell the doctor right then and there that you already did the scan and it shows 535mls. You can immediately get the order for the straight cath or foley and help your patient feel much better.

Those are just a few of the learning experiences I've encountered. Do yourself a favor and when you're on your new graduate preceptor ship, ask as many nurses as possible, especially your preceptor, if they have made any mistakes while contacting physicians. You may be surprised by the answers and also the nurses' willingness to share their bloopers.

In the last part of this chapter, I want to tell you about the emergency response teams most hospitals and patient care facilities have set up. They are all called different names, including MRTs or Medical Response Teams, RRTs or Rapid Response Teams and STAT teams. The bottom line is that these teams are designed for a few reasons. One of them being when you need a physician's input immediately and you're not getting a fast response from the patient's doctor. They also are designed to prevent a code blue from ever needing to be called.

Since this chapter is primarily focused on how to contact physicians, let's start there. Sometimes you have paged or called the physician and received no response. However, you really need to notify a physician so you can safely take care of your patient, and this isn't something that can wait any longer. That's when you would use an emergency response team. It is difficult to know what kind of situation calls for this type of intervention. Asking other experienced nurses and consulting your charge nurse are sometimes the best things to do to see if it is appropriate.

However, always remember, no matter what anyone says, it is your right to make this call anytime you think you may need to. When I first started out as a nurse, I made these types of calls all of the time. There were many times when I know I saved patient's lives because they were really going downhill fast. There were also a few times when the team didn't think anything severe was wrong and no new plans were made for the patient's care. That is also ok. This is just to get a second opinion, and it is better to be safe than sorry.

These teams are usually comprised of one or two ICU nurses, the nursing supervisor and the on-call physician. Additionally, when these calls are made, a phlebotomist often comes and many times an EKG technician also shows up. Your charge nurse should also hopefully be in the room with you, as well as another nurse or two from your unit.

These situations can be quite intimidating, especially for new nurses, because every time someone new shows up from the team, they are going to want to know from you what is going on. The first thing you need to tell them is why you made the call. Your patient had a seizure, or their blood pressure was critically high or low, or they looked like they were having difficulty breathing and their oxygen saturation was critical.

The next thing the team needs to know is your patient's history. This includes their admitting diagnosis; medical history; previous assessments done by you or if this is a new patient for you; what were you told in report; what medications have they had today and in the past; was there anything new that happened that could have possibly led to this situation, etc..

Then together as a team, it is time to see if any new test needs to be ordered or new medications need to be added or if the patient should be transferred to a different level of care. The reasons these teams were designed was to give nurses and family members a backup. You don't want to wait until your patient isn't breathing to call for help; if something just isn't right, call it. For me it is very comforting to know that even if I cannot reach the physician assigned to my patient, ultimately my patients will be taken care of.

Caroline Porter Thomas

Chapter 8

When and How to Review Labs

"Determine never to be idle. No person will have occasion to complain of the want of time who never loses any. It is wonderful how much may be done if we are always doing." – Thomas Jefferson

When I was in nursing school, I remembered learning so much about all of the labs, and then I basically forgot most of what I learned. I know I might hear some criticism from educators or other professional personnel, but I just want to be real with you. In nursing school, we learn a little about everything. But once you're working and depending on the specialty you work in, you'll learn the specific labs that are pertinent to your job.

Since I float to different units, I truly witness this firsthand. The other day I floated to a psychiatric unit. The only labs they checked on a frequent basis were the labs pertinent to detection of medication levels still in the blood. When I float to the intensive care units, I'm always amazed at how much more the nurses know regarding their patients' labs. When you work in your specialty, you'll learn what is important to that specialty.

The time to look at labs is hopefully first thing in the morning. I say hopefully because that is ideal. I've worked in a few hospitals where phlebotomy collects their non-stat routine labs around 8-9 a.m. This means the values wouldn't show until around 11ish. This was super

Caroline Porter Thomas

inconvenient and I would find myself forgetting to look at them because as the day gets later, you just have other things on your mind.

However, after working at that location awhile, I found that if I put a sticky note on my notebook that said 1100, I'd remember to check the labs. Hopefully the hospital or patient care facility that you get hired for does the nice thing and collects their labs very early. This way when you come in and get your assignment, you can quickly glance through and then be on your way.

As a Telemetry nurse, I quickly glace at about five-six different labs: the potassium level, the sodium level, the BUN & creatinine, the hematocrit and hemoglobin. Also, if they have cardiac enzymes drawn, CK & troponin. I quickly glance at all of the lab values and see if any are super high or super low.

Some of the lab values when out of range are easy to fix medically. The potassium level, for example, can easily be corrected. If it's low, a replacement can be given in tablets, liquid or IV form. If it's too high, Kayexalate can be given so it's excreted via the GI track.

If I'm unfamiliar with other lab values that may be out of range, I usually look at the doctor's notes and see if they're aware of it. If there is a note, I know they are taking care of it. If there is not a note, I will mention it to the doctor when they're on the unit.

One of the best things you can do while you're on your new graduate orientation is to converse with your preceptor and ask how and when he/she looks at the patient labs. Make this your routine as well. Someone who is experienced in your specialty and also was looked upon as successful enough to precept a new graduate will have the best advice.

Caroline Porter Thomas

Chapter 9

What to Ask in Report

"If you go looking for a friend, you're going to find they're scarce. If you go out to be a friend, you'll find them everywhere." – Zig Ziglar

The nursing handoff or report is a bit of an art. No two days will be identical. Every nurse, every patient, every unit has so much variety that no absolute routine will ever be established. Sometimes you can be done with report in 30 minutes, or it can take you 1 ½ hours. Sometimes you're lucky enough to get report from one nurse. Sometimes a different nurse will be assigned to every patient.

I'm not sure how it's going to be at your place of work, but nowadays in almost all of the facilities where I work, we do report in the room. Personally I like this; it's more time consuming, but I do believe it's safer. Let me explain how report was in the past so you can compare.

Previously, all the nurses would sit in the break room and the oncoming nurse would get verbal information concerning his/her patients from the previous shift nurse. What was bad about this is that there would be a lot of information shared in these rooms that was not necessary. Gossip about the patients was commonplace, which I personally could not stand. Also, there were many times I got report on my patient and then saw the patient, and thought, "Did the nurse tell me about the wrong patient?"

Caroline Porter Thomas

It was easy to forget about major things concerning the patient's care. I would often walk into my patient's room after report and notice that the patient had a wound vac on, or had IV fluid running or was on 3 liters of oxygen. These things are hard to miss when you're giving report in the room.

The other thing was that the patients were left completely out of the loop. The most important person who needs to know what is going on is the patient; if it were concerning you, you would want to know the plan as well. Giving report in the room helps your patients who are alert and oriented know more about what the day or night has in store for them.

Today, most likely, you will receive reports in the room. Let me share with you some tips on how to get all of the information that you need. First of all, you need to do the same thing every time. Basically, you must have a systematic approach. Depending on where you work, you may need to have your own sheet ready or the department may print out a sheet for you with your patient's general information. Some of the sheets also have room for you to document the assessment information you receive from the oncoming nurse, i.e., the neurologic information, respiratory information, so on and so forth.

This is the standard information you should already have: your patient's name, age, admitting diagnosis and the primary doctor. In report with the other nurse, they'll let you know if the patient has any previous medical history, allergies and any consulted specialty physicians (such as a gastroenterologist). In this report, you should also discuss what the patient's diet is and how they are tolerating it.

Next ask about the patient's activity level; here you want to know two things, what did the physician order and what is the patient capable of. Then ask about the IV, is it working (meaning you can flush saline through it); when it's working, many nurses will say that the IV is patent. After this, find out about any abnormal labs and vital signs.

Finally, you want a quick update about what the previous nurse found when doing their own physical assessment on the patient. Have a list of all the major systems so that you don't forget anything. Here are the eight major systems I ask about in my report: 1. Neurologic 2. EENT (Eyes, Ears, Nose, Throat) 3. Respiratory 4. Cardiac 5. Urinary 6. Gastrointestinal 7. Musculoskeletal 8. Integumentary.

Here is what I'm looking for:

1. Neurologic – are they alert and oriented X 4, are they calm and cooperative, any systemic neurologic problems?
2. EENT – Can they see fine, can they hear ok; the nose and throat I usually don't ask about.
3. Respiratory – How is their breathing, are they on oxygen, how did their lungs sound to you (previous nurse)?
4. Cardiac – How does their heart sound, do they have good pulses, any edema on any extremities?
5.   Urinary – How are they going to the bathroom? Do they get up and walk to the bathroom, do they use the urinal, when was the last time they voided?
6. Gastrointestinal – Does the patient have good bowel sounds and when was their last bowel movement?

7. Musculoskeletal – Can they walk, do they have tremors, are they steady, do they call when they need assistance? If bed bound and they need to be turned every two hours, how many people does it take to do this? If your patient is able to help you, sometimes you can help them turn by yourself. Otherwise, every single turn may take multiple people; knowing in advance will help you plan your day.

8. Integumentery – How does their skin look, do they have any open areas on their body, especially their sacrum if they are bed bound? If they need to be turned every two hours, when was the last time they were turned.

Your goal here is to get the previous nurse's findings so that when you do your own assessments, you'll be able to compare. Is your patient progressing? Hopefully, this is the case. However, if your patient is regressing, this is also very important to know. Doing the report in the room allows you to physically look at the patient while the nurse is giving you this information, just in case you need to clarify something.

You can use this time to clarify things only. It is not appropriate . . . or nice . . . to start doing your own assessment. Remember, the nurse who is giving you report has been there for the last 12, sometimes 13, hours, so let them quickly give their reports so they can go home. Also, I hope this goes without saying, but this gives the outgoing nurse a chance to day goodbye and introduce you the oncoming nurse.

At this time, it's very important that you quickly update the white board in your patient's room so they have your information and that of everyone involved in their care. I write down the charge nurse, their nursing assistant and, of course, my information. I also write down any numbers needed to reach us. Then I'm off to the next patient.

The only problems I do have with report in the room is that it is much more time consuming. Depending on your patient and their needs, many times you will walk into the room and they will need help going to the bathroom, or have multiple questions regarding their care. It is definitely good for your patients to be concerned and involved in their care but you have many patients to get report on. Reminding yourself that this is a good thing for your patient to be involved will help you stay calm and focused.

Another issue I have with in-the-room report is that unit directors are always trying to rush this process. I understand why, of course; when two sets of nurses are there, the hospital is paying for two nurses instead of one. There are a few things you can do speed up the process. Being ready on time is a big thing, and also let the outgoing nurse pass on things that are left to do easily. Remember that nursing is a 24/7 job and one day, you'll need to pass something on to the next nurse.

Always remember though, no matter how much people rush you to be faster, get the information you need to practice your job safely. That is why you need a systematic approach and to get all of your information the same way each time. As I mentioned before, your unit may give you a sheet for report; however, I have attached the sheet that I use when I do not receive this sheet so that you can use this one or design one of your own that works for you better.

Caroline Porter Thomas

Room# Pt. Name Dr. Name			
Diagnosis History			
Allergies			
Diet & Toleration			
Activity			
ACHS			
Meds/IV Site & fluids			
Abnormal labs	⊳—⟨ ⊣⊢⟨	⊳—⟨ ⊣⊢⟨	⊳—⟨ ⊣⊢⟨
Abnormal Vital Signs			
Abnormal Systems: Neurologic EENT Respiratory Cardiac Urinary Gastro Musculoskeletal Integumentary			
Notes:			

Note: I only write abnormal, so that I can quickly glance at this sheet and see where I need to pay special attention. Also, for symbols under lab section email me at Caroline@EmpoweRN.com

Since you are a new graduate there are going to be many words, abbreviations and sayings that you aren't familiar with. I remember so clearly being amazed when I first started and watched nurses give report. "She has a 20 in the right AC, with D5 1/2NS with 20 of K going at 50. The Chest X-Ray and CAT scan showed bilateral infiltrates so the pt. is also on antibiotics. The Nuc/Med test was negative for PE, room air sat was 91 so we have her on 2L, her K was 3.4 so she had a replacement of 40 PO..." The nurses would just go on and on in this different language, and the receiving nurse would understand everything.

I longed for the day when I could easily grasp the report information and understand everything the nurse was telling me. The fact is this: In nursing, we do the same things over and over. Experience is the only way to make the report easier and easier. You will hear the same sayings, abbreviations and situations repeatedly. Pretty soon, you will be able to easily glide through the report.

Until then, though, you have got to slow the fast nurses down. Some nurses will get upset when you ask them to slow down. Sometimes I guess they really could be in a hurry. However, you must always remember, safety first. Those two words that you didn't understand could have been very important concerning your patient's care. So I want you to play the "New Graduate Card."

When I first started taking report on my own, especially transfer reports on the phone (patients coming from different units to me), one of the first things I would say was, "Please go slow. I just graduated and this is one of the first times I'm taking report on my own." I did this for almost an entire year. If you are up front with nurses and tell them they need to go a little slow in the beginning because you're just starting out, usually they will be a little more sympathetic.

Also, never never feel stupid asking questions. At least once or twice a day EVERY single day while I am getting report, I ask "What is that?" or "What do I need to do for that?" I don't care if I look stupid. In fact, I would rather look stupid to the nurse I'm getting report from than make a mistake and look even more stupid in front of a much larger audience.

There are many times when I'm getting report that I ask, "Why did they give that medication?" or "Why did they perform that surgery?" or especially to the surgical or PACU nurses, "What was that procedure again???" Oftentimes, there are new medications introduced and this is how we find out . . . in report. Or surgeons or doctors start regularly performing new procedures or prescribing new medications. Asking questions is exactly how I become familiar with them.

Play the new graduate card as long as you need to. There is no time limit that says you can no longer say you're a new graduate. Use this also when you are giving report to another nurse. That will let them know that they need to be a little easy on you. Personally, I did this for at least a year. And I don't hesitate to pretend as if I'm new if someone giving me report is seriously talking too fast.

Chapter 10

How to Manage High Nurse to Patient Ratios

"If your actions inspire others to dream more, learn more, do more and become more, you are a leader." – John Quincy Adams

I remember like it was yesterday. We were short one nurse because her child was sick and our unit was extremely busy. I was already over the max load with one extra patient, making a total of six patients on an Intermediate Care Unit. New orders on all of my patients were streaming in, my phone kept ringing and ringing and every time I looked up I had a "Performance Improvement" personnel reminding me of something else I needed to do. I was quite literally overwhelmed.

Every nurse on our unit was the same; even our charge nurse who wasn't supposed to have any patients had four. We were all strung out and every nurse, even me, was talking about it. "How is this safe?" "I'm so busy I can't even think." "Why do they keep sending new patients?" "This is a great way for us to lose our licenses!"

And then, my limit was pushed. The charge nurse approached me with a graven face. "Caroline, you're the only nurse here that I know can handle this. You are going to get a seventh patient. The ER is full and they have patients waiting in the halls. We have one open bed on this unit and they are sending a patient now."

My patient came just as the charge nurse was telling me this. I didn't even have time to object. I stood there for a second, first insanely mad... why did I even want to be a nurse? I didn't know what to do. I seriously started to tear up. My mind was going a thousand miles a minute. I was so massively behind on all of my charting and medication administrations. And then, I had a breakthrough.

"Take a deep breath, Caroline," a voice inside me said. Quiet your mind, everything will work out. I realized when I was running around like crazy, complaining and letting my mind run like crazy... I wasn't breathing. This patient deserved my best care. I put my attention on my new patient. I went over and greeted him. I let go of all the reasons why he shouldn't be my patient, I let go of cursing the nursing staffing supervisors for sending me too much work. I just let go, breathed, quieted my mind and focused.

I focused on this beautiful person in front of me. I settled him into his room; I took his height, weight, vital signs. I asked him all of the admission questions. This patient had my complete attention. At that moment, I didn't feel like there was anything else more important in the entire world than this new patient.

This breakthrough carried over into my other patients. "What if I always say this to myself?" I asked. What if I believed that there was nothing more important than what I'm doing right now? What if I quiet my mind regularly by breathing deep and not speaking about the injustices I currently face?

And then I also thought about this. There is a bigger problem I could face. What if I didn't have any patients? I wouldn't have a job! I would not be able to use my skills, my license and my gifts! I would be home, doing nothing. At that moment, I decided to be different. I will no longer complain about heavy workloads. I will be grateful for the opportunity to serve.

I will be grateful every time I get a new patient because every person in the world deserves to be treated with the best care that I can give. Every time a nurse complains to me, I will not take the opportunity to tell him/her how hard my load is today too. I will not tell other nurses to not complain; I will only lead by example and not complain myself.

At this point, I realized that one of the hardest days of my life had turned into the greatest. I've always loved being a nurse. I love to help people and go the extra mile to put a smile on someone's face. But recently I had lost my edge. I had spent too much time sitting at the nursing station or nursing lounge listening to co-workers complain and joining into the conversation of negativity. I had stopped focusing on how hard I worked to be exactly where I am right now. I had stopped being grateful for every challenge that came my way.

With this new focus and clarity, I was able to take a step back and look at my patients and their care. I quickly evaluated what my next steps needed to be. I planned my course of action and got in the "zone." Task by task, I properly and elegantly cared for my more than heavy load. Because I knew I didn't have a lot of time to connect with all of my patients as I usually did, I made each second count.

I would look each patient directly in the eyes, making sure if appropriate that I had a smile on my face. If they were lying in the bed, I would kneel down to their eye level and ask if they needed anything or if they were ok. I made it a point to show them, through my body posture and eyes, that I cared and that they are important, and that I am here for them.

If they asked me a question, I would immediately take a deep breath in. What this did was first of all give me very necessary oxygen, but it also settled down the voice inside my head telling me about all the other things I needed to do. I wanted each of my patients to know that I was present and listening.

You see, many times, it's not how many patients we have or how much care they involve that gets us off kilter. It is the thoughts we choose to indulge in. Make no mistake, as a nurse there will be times you will get behind, or have a patient fall seriously, acutely ill, or have family members following you down the halls thinking you only have their mom as a patient. But how much more equipped to handle this would you be with a clear and focused mind?

I learned that day that this needs to be a priority for me every second of every day. I need to constantly ask myself, "How can I focus better?" "How can I serve better?" Asking these questions, I have come up with several answers. As you go along, you'll also come up with answers specific to you. The key is just to ask the questions all the time.

The first thing I learned on how to manage very high nurse/patient ratios is that I need to practice faith. I believe in God. I believe that I am created from love and that I need to be challenged frequently in order to be the person I need to be to serve better. I also believe that no matter what situation I face… I will ultimately be OK.

I used to worry constantly about making a terrifying mistake that would cost me my license. I would carry this fear along, thinking over and over about the stories I heard in nursing school or orientation or the break room. I would also worry about getting sued for not giving good care.

With faith, I turned this worry into thoughts of conquering and overcoming. I thought what if I gave such great, passionate and loving care that my patients remembered me until the day they died. What if my care was so amazing that they told the unit director about me? I then also focused on how little my part in the world is. I developed the belief that there is no ultimate mistake I can make that will ruin me. I am a survivor; I will learn and I will become better.

I want you to take this opportunity to get connected to yourself and your beliefs. Develop beliefs that empower you to be better. You have control over this. It's just a matter of exercising these thoughts and spiritual practices and applying them to your daily work. You can make your place of work the most Holy place in the world. You can grow from every mistake when you practice faith.

The next thing that I do to successfully manage high nurse/patient ratios is that I make sure I am taken care of. This may sound like common sense when you are reading this. We have heard all too often that you cannot take care of anyone else unless you take care of yourself. However, daily practice on the job is harder.

It is really easy to say to yourself, "I will do this really quickly and then eat a bite of something." I see so many nurses (and I used to do it too) who would literally work themselves to death. Guys, it is not heroic to go seven hours without eating, drinking or using the bathroom. I once worked with a nurse who would chew gum the entire 12 hours so that she wouldn't get thirsty, drink and have to waste time to go to the bathroom. That is crazy!

The real art is to learn how to care for yourself AND all of your patients. There are several ways I do this and it does involve a lot of pre-planning… especially with food. I will discuss exactly how and what I bring with me to eat every day. But just know that if you are hungry, it's hard to focus. Just a few bites of something can take that feeling away and you have your focus back. It is also really difficult to completely focus if you have to go the bathroom. Just do your business quickly and get back out there!

Always ask yourself how you can feel better on the job. Make this a priority. The better you feel, the better you will be able to help your patients feel good. Listen to your body's needs. Make yourself the most important person in the world. If you don't, who will? By understanding how it is to be well taken care of, you will be able to spread an immense amount of love to all of the people you come in contact with.

The next thing that helps me have complete focus is ensuring my environment is neat and clean. I make sure my notebook is organized, that my sticky notes are aligned, that my writing is neat. As much as possible, I make sure my patients' rooms are neat, that all of the trash is in the trash can, that everything possible is in the drawers. To me, a cluttered outside, means a cluttered mind, which ultimately means less focus and worse patient care. I make it a point to clean and pick up frequently.

Walking fast is another thing I love to do that helps me manage so many patients. I find it very therapeutic. I love racing down the halls and trying to beat my pace constantly. Sometimes I move so fast that other nurses ask me if I'm OK because I'm so rushed; it's kind of funny. But I absolutely love how we move so much in this profession. I honestly do not know how people can stand desk jobs. I get depressed thinking about sitting all day.

I also love how Dr. Oz emphasizes that we should walk at least 5 miles a day. That is almost always a piece of cake as a nurse! I used to wear a pedometer regularly, and I found out that I walk at least that much. Sometimes on really busy days, I walk way more. It really is a blessing to have a job where we are so active.

As I walk down the halls, in order to maintain a clear and focused mind, I take very deep breaths and count up to 6. When I breathe out, I do the same, count to 6. So as you're walking in and out of patient rooms, performing care, make sure you pick up your pace and make it a point to stay moving all the time.

The last piece of advice I want to give you to give awesome patient care to lots of patients is to "get your hands dirty." What I mean by that is to get in the "Just do it mode." If your patient asks you for the bed pan, just do it, right then, right there. Don't go looking around for the

Caroline Porter Thomas

nursing assistant every time. There will be times when that it is necessary, but definitely not every time.

Don't look for ways to get out of work. Just get in the "I will do it!" mode. If you notice that your total care patient smells less than fresh, check right then, right there. If you need a set of vital signs, do it. If your patient's food needs to be warmed up, do it. Look, there is a time for delegation and asking for help.

However, if you just get in the mind set that you are here to serve in any and every way possible, you will not need to spend wasted time looking for help. Also, be mindful of all the patients on the floor; if another nurse's patient needs help to the bathroom, help them. And trust me, when you do need something, everyone around you will bend over backwards to help you.

Chapter 11

How to Handle Constant New Responsibilities

"The three great essentials to achieve anything worthwhile are, first, hard work; second, stick-to-itiveness; third, common sense."

— *Thomas A. Edison*

For me, it is always easy to know when new tasks have been assigned to our already busy lives as nurses. The way I can tell is the level of complaints in the break room. In the mornings, I do my best to just get in and get out as quick as possible; however, sometimes the complaints are so loud and unanimous that they are difficult to ignore.

I've often wondered why people in general spend their time and priceless energy complaining about things that they cannot change. I also wonder why they create images in their heads that disempower them, but aren't based on truth. I hear people saying things like, "There are too many people just sitting there in the corner office thinking of new ways to keep us busy." Take a second and visualize that.

Let's even exaggerate a little if you will. So here we have it. An older man, white hair wearing a nice suit, sitting in his corner office. He has his hands folded on his belly and his feet up on the desk. He has TV screens all around him where he watches his hospital employees and thinks of new things to make them do so that they are busy. Does this image empower or aggravate you? The words you use and the metaphors you create give you energy or take energy away.

What if you create a new vision that helps you understand why the new responsibilities are being added? None of this is based on truth, so play with it a little. What if instead of the older man relaxing in the chair you create an image of a team of very hard working men and women who have just gotten statistics back on the project they were assigned to work on?

Those stats showed that some hospitals made changes and got lower hospital-acquired infection rates. In fact, what if this rate was so dramatically different that their bosses sent them emails and called them saying that changes had to be made or else their jobs were on the line. So they scurried around trying to develop the easiest way to implement this process. They work tirelessly to find ways to make it easier on their already overworked staff, but to also meet the requirements that have proven results.

Then after much thought, contemplation, research and careful evaluations, the new responsibility is released. After which, floods of emails complaining about the new task swamp their computers. They receive emails from unit directors saying that the task is too much for the staff to do and to see if they can find ways to make it easier. They receive emails from the staff accusing them of having nothing better to do than make their jobs harder. Then they also receive emails from their bosses who are also receiving complaint emails. Their bosses want to know why they didn't find ways to make it easier for the staff to assimilate.

You see, neither of these metaphors are based on reality. However, in the first one about the older man, you felt kind of like an overworked puppet. In the second one, though, you could see how there were hardworking people analyzing data and carefully considering the best way to make your place of work safer. They are real people with feelings and lots of pressure placed on them.

Listen, I've been a nurse for about five years. I've had my share of new responsibilities added to the table. Let me share with you a few of them and how I've still been able to love my job.

The first is the rounding sheet. Now that HCAHPS plays a major role in reimbursement, hospital directors are on their staff about ways to make their score higher and higher. Nurses have a lot to do with these scores because we are the ones with the patients the most. So what is the HCAHPS? On the top of their website it says "Hospital Care Quality Information from the Consumer Perspective."

Basically, it involves a series of questions designed to figure out the patients' perception of the care they received at your hospital. When patients go home, they receive a telephone call or a survey questionnaire in the mail asking them specific questions about their recent hospital visit. From the answers that are provided, each hospital is given a score based on a certain number of questionnaires filled out. The higher the score the better, and vice versa.

Here are the questions taken directly from the HCAHPSonline.org. Familiarize yourself with these questions now and it will make your life a little easier later:

Your Care from Nurses:
1. During this hospital stay, how often did nurses treat you with courtesy and respect?
    1. Never
    2. Sometimes
    3. Usually
    4. Always

2. During this hospital stay, how often did nurses listen carefully to you?
    1. Never
    2. Sometimes
    3. Usually
    4. Always

3. During this hospital stay, how often did nurses explain things in a way you could understand?
    1. Never
    2. Sometimes
    3. Usually
    4. Always

4. During this hospital stay, after you pressed the call button, how often did you get help as soon as you wanted it?
    1. Never
    2. Sometimes

3. Usually

4. Always

5. I never pressed the call button

Your Care from Doctors:

5. During this hospital stay, how often did doctors treat you with courtesy and respect?

1. Never

2. Sometimes

3. Usually

4. Always

6. During this hospital stay, how often did doctors listen carefully to you?

1. Never

2. Sometimes

3. Usually

4. Always

7. During this hospital stay, how often did doctors explain things in a way you could understand?

1. Never

2. Sometimes

3. Usually

4. Always

The Hospital Environment:

8. During this hospital stay, how often were your room and bathroom kept clean?

1. Never

2. Sometimes

3. Usually

4. Always

Caroline Porter Thomas

9. During this hospital stay, how often was the area around your room quiet at night?
   1. Never
   2. Sometimes
   3. Usually
   4. Always

Your Experiences in This Hospital
10. During this hospital stay, did you need help from the nurses or other hospital staff in getting to the bathroom or in using a bedpan?
   1. Yes
   2. No -> if No, Go the Question 12

11. How often did you get help in getting to the bathroom or in using bedpan as soon as you wanted?
   1. Never
   2. Sometimes
   3. Usually
   4. Always

12. During this hospital stay, did you need medicine for pain?
   1. Yes
   2. No -> If N, Go to Question 15

13. During this hospital stay, how often was your pain well controlled?
   1. Never
   2. Sometimes
   3. Usually
   4. Always

14. During this hospital stay, how often did the hospital staff do everything they could to help you with your pain?

1. Never
2. Sometimes
3. Usually
4. Always

15. During this hospital stay, were you given any medicine that you had not taken before?
1. Yes
2. No -> if No, Go to question 18

16. Before giving you any new medicine, how often did the hospital staff tell you what the medicine was for?
1. Never
2. Sometimes
3. Usually
4. Always

17. Before giving you any new medicine, how often did hospital staff describe possible side effects in a way you could understand?
1. Never
2. Sometimes
3. Usually
4. Always

When You Left the Hospital:

18. After you left the hospital, did you go directly to your own home, to someone else's home, or to another health facility?
1. Own home
2. Someone else's home
3. Another health facility -> go to question 21

19. During this hospital stay, did doctors, nurses or other hospital staff talk with you about whether you would have the help you needed when you left the hospital?
    1. Yes
    2. No

20. During this hospital stay, did you get information in writing about what symptoms or health problems to look out for after you left the hospital?
    1. Yes
    2. No

Overall Rating of Hospital

21. Using any number from 0 to 10, where 0 is the worst hospital possible and 10 is the best hospital possible, what number would you use to rate this hospital during your stay?

22. Would you recommend this hospital to your friends and family?
    1. Definitely no
    2. Probably no
    3. Probably yes
    4. Definitely yes

There are two reasons I took the time to type these questions out word for word from the HCAHPS website. The first is because this is where the majority of our new responsibilities are coming from. Each hospital receives a score and from this score they see the exact areas that we need to improve on.

I spoke earlier about the new responsibility of the hourly rounding sign in sheet. The reason that many unit directors are choosing to use this is because if you regularly round on your patients, you are obviously with them more.

The more you are with them, the more likely they are to trust you and ask questions to clarify things they don't know.

The second reason that I took the time to type out all of the questions is because I wanted you to notice something. Even though the first section says "Care from your Nurses," did you notice that many of the other questions involve nurses as well? For example, the question that asks about meeting bathroom needs. Also, the question about pain management. In general, nurses have more responsibility for the HCAHPS score than any other department in the hospital.

What I have realized is that one way to embrace new responsibilities is to understand the root of their creation. The more you understand the reason, the more likely you are to accept the new task without anger. Believe me, sometimes it is easier than others to do this. Let me tell you quickly a few experiences I've had so you can see how quickly things can change.

One busy day when we were short staffed and I had six patients on an IMCU (InterMediate Care Unit), I got a phone call from our unit pharmacist. "You are taking care of 404-1, 406-1 and 406-2, right?" she asked. I told her that was correct. "Well, they have all responded that they would like the influenza vaccine." I was really confused at this point. We always gave the influenza vaccine right before the patients were discharged. Why was she calling me about this?

She explained, "Our policy has changed and we are now giving the influenza vaccines upon admission. Too many vaccinations were being missed. Now it is the admitting nurse's responsibility to give the vaccine, and if he/she cannot they need to write a note explaining and then also document that they have passed it on to the next nurse. Since the admitting nurses didn't do this last night, it is your responsibility to give these patients their vaccines now."

Right this second? I thought. I don't exactly remember what I was dealing with that day, but I can remember thinking; "Influenza vaccines are the least of my worries at this second." So my first reaction was to be upset about it. It is, after all, more work to my already heavy load.

It was not until a few weeks later, though, that I witnessed my first patient spiral downward from influenza. Terrible, isn't it, how sometimes we need real experiences to help us understand how important things are? I watched my poor patient get completely worn out from fighting this illness. His face was beet red from a very high fever, and he couldn't stop coughing; he had tears in his eyes from a headache that no medications were helping. Then he started having difficulty breathing. I had to call for help at that point.

"Ok," I thought, I learned my lesson. This is an important task that we need to just do as soon as possible. From that point on, I immediately gave each patient who agreed the vaccination. This was one real life example of how new responsibilities were added and then I was able to clinically see the necessity.

There are going to constantly be new, added responsibilities. Knowing that will help you anticipate new tasks. The best thing you can do is to take Nike's advice and without question, JUST DO IT. It does not change anything if you add to the noise level in the break room. It will just get you worked up for nothing.

If you need any help finding an empowering reason behind a new task added to your list, email me at Caroline@EmpoweRN.com and we can work through this together.

Chapter 12

How to Establish Yourself as a Team Player

"Coming together is a beginning, staying together is progress, and working together is success." Henry Ford

As a nurse, there really is no way to complete your tasks all the time without the help of your coworkers. There will be times when one patient requires too much care for you to handle alone. This can be in the form of medical necessity and also some people, in general, demand more care than others. Patients, assignments and workloads will be different every single day. You never know when the day will come when you will need to rely a lot on your co-workers.

Let me tell you a story of when I desperately needed my co-workers and these beautiful ladies and gentlemen came through in a great way. One day it seemed as though I had very critically sick patients. On an IMCU unit, this isn't uncommon; however, usually there are only one or two patients who I really feel as if I have to keep very close eyes on. That day, though, there were three who I was concerned about. The unit was already short a nurse and I had six patients. All of the nurses really were extremely busy themselves.

I started my day, getting report and then doing vital signs and assessments. I have learned that it's best to attack your work in the morning and move super fast. I started by getting my patients' temperatures and talking to them while I applied the pulse OX and BP cuff. While I waited for the BP, I listened to my patients' lungs, heart and then I palpated and listened to their abdomens. I quickly go down to the legs and check for edema and, from that point, I ask if they have any sores or open areas on their body and ask if I can quickly check their skin. This takes seriously 3 minutes once the routine is down.

Right after this, I mean standing right there, I documented everything. The vital signs, the assessment and everything else that is required, i.e.. the Falls score, the pressure sore risk. This usually took another 3 minutes of total focus. I usually finished everything in about 6 minutes and then it was on to the next! This day, however, I was so worried and stressed about the acuity of my patients that I was moving even faster. Literally finishing everything in like 4 minutes.

Then, when I was about half-way through this morning routine, I got a call from the secretary. "Your patient's husband in room 305 came out and said his wife was having a stroke." I was so confused. I was deep in thought from my morning routine flow and she was one of the patients I had just assessed literally 15 minutes ago. I headed to the room, and before I even arrived, I heard a Medical Response Team being called to that room.

I entered to find one of my co-workers already getting vital signs and doing neuro checks. My co-worker had seen my patient's husband in the hall and had gone into the room to assess my patient. When you think about this, it was a very nice thing for him to do. I'm sure with his workload that he also was pretty behind his work, as well. When the emergency call was made, even more of my co-workers came to see if they could help. What really surprised me, though, was when one of them asked me if there was any help I needed with any of my other patients. What a thoughtful question.

It was one of the most thoughtful questions that I had ever heard. I mean, think about it. When an emergency is called, it is everyone's nature to want to see what is going on. The weirder and more gruesome it is, the more people will show up. I have to admit that has been my own response many times. You hear an emergency called and you rush to see what all the fuss is about. This part of our human nature has kept the news companies in business for many years.

They constantly show clips of the most disastrous and terrible things that have happened across the world, and we are glued to the TV, spurred by our human feeling of having to know. When I got a ton of help when my patient was declining, it was nice. But one nurse went over the top and taught me a great lesson in teamwork that I remember to this day. In fact, this is the main question that I try to ask when a nurse does have an emergency.

An emergency like this can take a lot of time. A typical emergency call, especially if the patient is transferred to another unit, can literally take 30 minutes to 1 hour. Can you imagine that much time taken out of your day, especially in the morning? You can be behind on your medication administration and assessments and with new orders constantly coming in . . . it can be overwhelming.

Many nurses you will see just sit at the desk and chat when they are caught up. Sometimes you'll walk around like a chicken with its head cut off and they will not notice, or if they notice, they still won't ask if you need help. When someone does take notice and offers to give you a hand, it is really nice. I've learned to watch for nurses who may look like they are in crisis and see if I can offer to help them with anything.

This is a great way to gain rapport with the nurses on the unit. Listen, guys, our job is so much harder than most jobs. I find myself saying, "Wow, I never thought I could do so much in one day" all the time. The number of patients we take, the amount of medications we give, the dressing changes, the talking to patients to make sure they are happy. All of this takes tons of time and, if you see a nurse really drowning, lend a hand. Even if it's to feed or turn his/her patient.

I want to tell you another story of what I have been through so you'll find ways to make it easier on everyone. One time I was getting report on a patient who had been on the unit for two weeks. Every nurse on the unit had this patient, so everyone was relieved that I was floating there to give the staff a break. The patient was fine, but the challenge was that her entire backside was a bedsore.

I guess the patient had been bed bound for quite some time and was initially at home and refused to turn; she developed a huge pressure sore. It was so bad that it was from her right to left hip and all the way down to each thigh. Exact measurements were nearly impossible and the wound therapy team spent two hours doing the best they could do. Her daily care, however, was to perform dressing changes BID or twice a day.

I heard in report that every time the dressing change needed to be done it took five nurses and at least 45 minutes. "Holy cow!" I thought. How on earth am I going to get almost all of the nurses on the unit to come in this room for an hour? Then I thought to myself, I wonder if they pre-planned and had everything ready. I thought some more and decided that the slowest time would be 2 p.m. This is usually when everyone is done with their assessments, medications and after most of the doctors have made their rounds.

So I asked every nurse on the unit personally if they could be in room 333 at 2 p.m. I also thought, well what would need to happen in order for a dressing change to go very fast? And then I planned to have all of the dressing material open, laid out and ready to go. I would even have the tape already torn in strips hanging from the bedside table and ready to go.

I then spoke to another nurse on the unit and asked her why this dressing change takes so long? He mentioned that nothing was ever ready when he got there, which I thought may have been one of the problems. Then he also said they give the patient a bath at the same time because it is the only time the patient will allow it.

This was great information because I knew exactly what I needed to do to help this flow better. In the past, I realized that even if you have a patient that you can't bathe by yourself, let's say for size purposes, that does not mean that you need help the entire time. In fact, you can completely wash the patient's front side, have it dried and even sometimes have the fresh gown on. After that you can ask someone for assistance and then wash their backside and change the sheets.

If you bathe your patients that way, it will make it a lot easier on your co-workers. Many times, when another nurse has asked me to help her with a bath, I go into the room and the water isn't even running. I try not to judge, but when you have a lot of other things to do, it's hard not to.

Also, I know many of you may be saying to yourselves, "It's not my job to bath my patients." Listen, everything the nursing assistant does is basically your responsibility. If your vital signs, blood sugars and basic patient care are not done by the nursing assistant, the next line of defense is you. The best nurses that I see have no clear definition of their jobs; they just do what needs to be done. You will never hear them say, "That's not my patient" or "That's not my job." They just do the work quietly and, honestly, joyfully. Get in the get-it-done attitude.

After he said that bathing the patient was one of the reasons it was taking so long, I knew what else I could do. I laid one more tangent to this question "What else can I do?" This question by the way, has led me to many answers that have helped me develop ways to make my job easier. Before I enter any room I ask the question, "What else can I do?" then, I ask myself questions like: has this patient asked for anything like juice or water, will I need to change linen, is there anything else that could make my patient's stay more comfortable? Secretly, I pretend that I work in a hotel in Japan.

Why Japan, you may ask. My husband and I went there for one of his conferences and they blew us away with their service and cheerful attitudes. When we arrived at the hotel, we were greeted by a beautiful Japanese woman with a warm smile and a bow. Yes, she literally bowed to us. At first, I thought it was weird. But since it was from the heart, I started to like it. It is part of their culture; she wasn't giving me special treatment or anything. You could just tell she was happy doing what she was doing.

Our stay at the hotel was awesome. Any time we needed anything, they went out of their way to do it or bring it, and fast. You could see how hard working each person was; they were extremely busy, but never too busy to give you their full attention. Any time you said thank you, they responded, "It was my pleasure." And I really believed them. So this is what I think about when I give care.

This is also how I find ways to make the dressing change easier for everyone… just by asking "What else can I do?" and thinking about how I can serve with pleasure. Once I decided that I would have everything ready and also have my patient's front side squeaky clean, can you imagine what happened at 2 p.m.? No one showed up in the room. I called the front desk and asked the secretary to call the nurses overhead. Finally two nurses showed up and I said, "Let's just see what we can do."

Would you believe that with my pre-planning and washing the patient's front side it took us less than 20 minutes? In the past, it took twice the staff and twice the time. Part of teamwork is being a good team player yourself. You have to understand that you are working with very busy people in a very busy environment. The more respectful you can be with their time, the better.

There are limits to what people can help you with. No one can document and assess for you. Also, it's not really fair to ask someone to do a dressing change for you because you have 12 hours to complete the task. The things that people can help you do are things like starting IV's, turning/changing your patient or giving a medication.

After years of being a nurse, I've realized that there are certain ways I can do things that make my life easier. I'm the type of person who likes to get my work done ASAP. With that said, I've also realized you cannot plan how your day is going to go. I mentioned earlier that I get my vital signs and document my assessments first thing in the morning. Many nurses will tell you not to worry about doing this now because you have 12 hours to complete it. For me, it hangs over my head like a cloud until it's done.

I do my documentation first thing for a very specific reason. There have been times, like the first story I told you, when early morning emergencies put me massively behind. It's one thing to be behind in your medications. But it is a really bad feeling when you have assessments AND medications to give AND then the discharges start to come in.

For some reason, just having those assessments documented first thing in the morning will help your day go much smoother. Now you have to be fast at this, really fast. Your goal as a new graduate will be to learn how to use the computer system quickly and accurately.

When you complete assessments early, you'll be clear on what is left to do. The medications ordered for your patient are something that every nurse on the unit can have access to if they just add that patient to their list. If you are behind and someone asks you if you need help, you could clearly say to them, "Please give room 555 her morning medications. I've already documented her vital signs and she wanted some Tylenol to go along with her morning medications for joint pain." This is a clear, concise request that should be relatively easy for another nurse to fulfill.

As a new graduate I know that you'll be a little more nervous about helping other nurses out, mainly because you feel as if you are the one who needs help the most. You can still develop great teamwork rapport with the nurses just by doing the little things. For example, feeding a patient, changing a patient, giving something for pain, taking a patient a snack, blanket or water. There is never a short list of things that you can help with. Also, in order to learn more, you could ask the nurse you are helping to call you if she has anything new or exciting that you could learn from.

When I was a new graduate, I realized the more experiences I had with my preceptor, the better. The only problem was that we had a certain number of patients and there were many days that I didn't learn anything new. I realized that just because there was nothing going on with my patients, that didn't mean there wasn't something going on with someone's patients.

I realized it was a lot of work to teach me something, which I guess is why a preceptor is assigned to new nurses. If I asked to watch a dressing change or bedside procedure with another nurse on the unit, they weren't always happy about it because that meant that they had to explain the procedure to me instead of just doing it.

In order to make it valuable for them to have me there, I made sure I was eager and helpful. I would be very attentive to ways I could help out before, during and after the procedure. I asked questions quickly, but if I didn't understand their rationale, I'd jot down a little note and then ask my preceptor for clarification.

The main thing I did even before knowing which nurse would have something going on was to plant the kindness seeds. Asking each nurse if they needed help with anything and being eager to help made most of the nurses on the unit willing to help me learn by teaching me a new skill.

Make sure you are open and eager to help everyone around you. Look for nurses on your unit who appear stressed out. This can be in the form of walking down the halls fast, a worried expression on his or her face, breathing heavily and complaining about too much work – you know the signs of being stressed out. Just pay attention and make it a priority to see how you can help.

I do have to say, because we cannot survive without each other, that helping out other nurses, helped me see many styles of nursing. There are nurses who you will ask for help and, while sitting down talking to another nurse, they will tell you they are too busy. There are other nurses who you will ask that you know are extremely busy and yet they'll drop whatever they're doing to lend you a hand.

In this situation, do your best not to judge the nurse who was sitting down and talking. Many people who say they are busy but do not appear to be busy may be overwhelmed in their heads. I've heard many nurses talk and they talk about how this is not good and that is not good and they basically overfill their minds to the point where they aren't really present. They seem to be unable to grasp the reality of what is happening right here and right now.

Use this as a lesson instead and focus on how absolutely amazing it was that the super busy nurse lent you a hand when you knew she didn't have a second to spare. What was going through that nurse's mind? How can you have that kind of attitude? Use these experiences

Caroline Porter Thomas

as a guide on what to do or not to do. In general, you can learn so much about time efficiency on this job by watching and learning from people who do a great job at it.

My final advice on how to have great teamwork with other nurses is to remind yourself constantly that you are here to serve. That means serving everyone around you, not just your patients. Think of yourself as here for the unit and every person who you are blessed to encounter throughout this day.

Chapter 13

How to Work as a Team with Your Nursing Assistants

"Life has taught us that love does not consist in gazing at each other, but in looking outward together in the same direction." – Antoine de Saint-Exupery

The nursing assistants are some of the most important individuals with whom you should make it a point to gain rapport. This group of individuals can really help you by making your job easier. However, if you have failed to develop a great relationship with them, they may avoid you like the plague and make your job much harder. The nursing assistant job, if done right, can be one of the most physically demanding jobs around so keep that in mind as you work.

When you are new to a unit, you want to establish the reputation of being a team player and hard worker. There is no room in the hospital for people who do not want to at least pull their own weight. The harder you work to do an exceptional job, the more respect you'll gain from those around you, including the nursing assistant. There are a few things you should know about their role so to be sensitive when asking for something.

First, understand what they are there for. Their most important task is patient daily care. Whether this is daily/nightly or checking and changing incontinent patients, their most important role is to assist the patient in being fresh and clean. This is especially important for patient comfort and also for our HCAHPS score. Believe me, if a family member walks in who has a mother or father who is bed bound for one reason or another, the first thing they are going to do is pull back the sheets and make sure their loved one has been attended to.

When you understand that your main concerns are different than their main concerns, you can adjust your daily plan accordingly. I oftentimes hear nurses complain that the nursing assistant forgot to recheck a patient's blood pressure after a medication was given. Understand that you are the one who is more concerned with the blood pressure because you can do something about it. And, honestly, I believe that is ok. We need different people to be concerned with different aspects of our patients so that as a whole, we can give the most complete care.

There have been many times when I myself have been very concerned and preoccupied with my patient's high or low blood pressure. There have also been way too many times when I've spent countless hours trying to notify a physician of my patient's positive blood cultures or low potassium. These are tasks that concern us as nurses, but they really don't affect our assistants, and rightly so. I can remember being busy doing these sorts of tasks and being relieved to see that my patient was given a bath, sheets changed and morning care attended to.

My patient had a warm, big smile on her face and it wasn't because I finally got a hold of the doctor to tell him about the critical magnesium level. Of course, the opposite has also been true. When I've been crazy busy and not had a chance to check on my patient, only to find out that no assistants had the chance, as well. In these times, it's best to just take immediate action and find ways to do what needs to be done right now. I will talk more on this at the end of the chapter.

When you get your assignment in the morning, take an additional second to find out what your assistants are going to be assigned, as well. You can find out a lot about how your day is going to go by knowing what they are going through. Did one nursing assistant not show up and there are three on the unit instead of four? Are they short staffed and each nursing assistant will be caring for 14 to 16 patients on the IMCU unit with many bed-bound patients?

Knowing what a reasonable number of patients is for nursing assistants on your particular unit is important. Because I usually work Tele or IMCU, I love it when I hear that my assistants have nine to 10 patients each. I believe that, for the most part, they should be able to stay on top of their patients or tasks. Of course, this does depend on the patients they are assigned. Sometimes you can have one patient who requires a lot of care from your assistant.

Knowing the number and type of patients assigned will help you be more sensitive when asking for help. Is your nursing assistant completely overwhelmed with jobs to do? Maybe this is not the best time to see if they can recheck a blood sugar. Ultimately, always remember that you are responsible for your patient's medical care and safety. Again, your nursing assistant's main concern should be bedside care.

Also understand that certain nursing assistant tasks can be much more time consuming than other tasks. For example, have you ever fed someone before? Sometimes this task alone can take 30 minutes for one patient. So if a nursing assistant tells you that they have three patients who need to be fed, realize that around mealtimes they are going to be pretty busy.

So how do you establish from the get-go that you are a team player? It's easy. You just do what needs to be done with or without your assistant's help. Remember, there are no clear roles in the hospital; however, we have one main goal and that is for safe, effective care given to uplift and heal our patients. For example, you notice that your incontinent patient is less than fresh, and if you are capable of changing them yourself, just do it!

Also, understand that every person is different and even though every nursing assistant essentially has about the same role, some handle the responsibility better than others. Some buckle under the pressure of increased work and others step up and tackle it. There is no right or wrong, really, but it's just a difference in personality. There are some nursing assistants who I have worked with that amazed me in their ability to multitask and take serious action.

I've worked in many hospitals now but, if you don't mind, I want to send a shout out to a few of them. From Central Carolina Hospital, Brenda and Nancy from the 3rd floor were so amazing and hardworking, thank you! Also from Holy Cross Hospital, the stars who stand out are Isatu from IMC and Fatuo from PCU. I love you both and enjoyed watching you give beautiful care. I have worked with many more amazing people but these are a few that are really on my mind.

Now, there will definitely be times when you work with assistants who you're sure are there to make your life a living nightmare. You'll need help badly. You'll be up to your head and completely overwhelmed with responsibilities. You may have patients who are going downhill fast. On top of that, you have other patients who you haven't been able to even see yet due to these critically ill patients.

Sometimes you won't be able to get the help you desperately need. It can make you feel as if you're all alone on the job. You may feel as if no one cares how hard you are working or what you have thus far accomplished. You may say something to the charge nurse about the aide's neglect and their attention is quickly diverted to other people with bigger problems.

Believe me; you'll have times like this. You may despise the people you are working with and even the profession you have chosen. When this happens, I believe it is most helpful to become present. What do I mean by that? Well, when we are busy and stressed out, our imaginations usually take over and all we see is the worst-case scenario.

We haven't been able to check on our patient in two hours, so we quickly see an image of the worst possible scenario. A picture flashes through your mind of your patient lying helplessly on the floor, crying out and wondering where you've been. You may also quickly see an image of all of your patients' faces with mad expressions on them. Or you may quickly see an image of yourself completely drowning on the job.

The first thing you need to do in this situation is take a deep breath and bring yourself back to reality. The quickest and most effective way that I find myself coming back to my senses is to find ways to feel like I am present and out of my crazy imagination. I will keep taking deep breaths and look at the facts. By doing this, I'll note the time and do a quick glance at all of my patients confirming that my imagination was dead wrong. Not one of my patients is on the floor and most of them seem relatively ok.

Then I will literally take two minutes and plan my course of action. Since asking my assistant for help is not an option, I'll look for other ways to perform my job. I ask other nurses for help all the time. Just getting a task done helps me breathe easier, and that's better than nagging my assistant every 10 minutes until he/she doesn't answer my telephone calls.

The other thing that I do that helps me stay in a loving and non-judgmental mindset is to develop the belief that people are doing the best they can with the resources they have available to them. This sentence was developed by Richard Bandler and John Grinder, a psychologist and linguist, respectively. They said that if you really took the time to judge why people do what they do, they always have a reason to back it up.

The point is that you never know what people are going through. You may think that your nursing assistant is completely ignoring you, when in reality she has two patients calling her every 10 minutes needing the bed pan or help to the toilette. Just having the overall belief that they are doing the best they can, will help you stay in a loving mindset. It's important that you have this belief, no matter how it looks on the outside. I've found that, in general, the people working in hospitals are really beautiful people deep inside and the more you can see that side of them, the better it is for you.

Chapter 14

How to Connect with Your Patients

"It really boils down to this: that all life is interrelated. We are all caught in an inescapable network of mutuality, tired into a single garment of destiny. Whatever affects one destiny, affects all indirectly."

— *Martin Luther King, Jr.*

Honestly, it seems almost silly for me to even think about writing a chapter about how to connect with your patients. Most people are drawn to nursing for this very reason. When I was in nursing school, we were asked why we wanted to be nurses and almost every single person in one form or another mentioned how they wanted to help people. What I have found, though, is that during the stress and business of our jobs, it's easy to forget the importance of minor shifts in our social approach to our patients. If these approaches are shifted slightly, our reason for being a nurse can come back with way more passion than before.

What I want to focus on in this chapter is very minor and seemingly insignificant behavior shifts that make all the difference. I cannot add time to your day; however, connection happens in an instant and honestly, more time will not even matter. What we need to focus on are ways to utilize our NET time or No Extra Time. This is what my hero, motivational speaker and author Tony Robbins, focuses on. What this means is changing the way we use the time we have that will help us maximize the impact.

Caroline Porter Thomas

Albert Mehrabian is a great psychologist who did a lot of research on communication, and he found that many factors are involved. What was really astounding, though, was that words convey only 7% of our message. Instinctively, you know this. If someone says they love you but in a tone and with body language that suggests otherwise, you get the message. If you apply this research to the way you carry out your nursing care, you'll be able to connect with almost every patient you have.

So if words are only 7%, what is the other 93%? Believe it or not, the tone in which you say something carries 38% of the message that you are trying to portray. The rest and majority of our message, 55%, is given through non-verbal behaviors, like body language, facial expressions or body movements. Knowing this, I make sure that using the little time that I have I engage all three of these behaviors for maximum impact of the message I need to get across.

If one of the tasks that I need to do for my job is to help my patient go to the bathroom, I want them to feel like they have all of the time in the world, even though this is not the case and I literally may have 10 REALLY important things that need to be done at that second. Using this knowledge, I can connect with my patient and make them feel comfortable.

When they ask for help, I verbally say "Of course." I watch my tone and body language to make sure that my message is congruent with my words. I make sure that I make eye contact with my patient while he/she asks me the question. One problem I sometimes encounter is that the little voice in my head is louder than my patient's voice. In order to quiet this little voice, I take a nice deep breath while looking at my patient. This helps me hear his/her voice much better.

Here are five behaviors I focus on constantly to make sure I am able to connect with my patients and be of best service. The first is to smile. When was the last time you were greeted by a nice warm smile? There is so much comfort when you see a face that is calm and filled with joy. Always remember, most people in the hospital would not be there if they had a choice. It is a very scary place and we as nurses and much of the hospital staff do very foreign and many times physically painful procedures. Many times, just a welcoming smile can make your patient forget about the pain they just endured.

Make it a point to make your face calm and approachable. It doesn't take 5 minutes for a smile to successfully form on your face. This important facial feature happens in an instant and is the most important item for you to focus on. This is using NET time in a way that will help you be more efficient and successful. You already have some type of expression on your face; make sure it is one that will help you and your patients.

Also, have you ever heard someone say the phrase, "You have to fake it before you make it"? There is much truth in this silly sentence. When you're genuinely smiling, it is impossible to be upset. That's why a smile equates to our brains as "Happiness." Because a person who is happy has a different expression than one who is upset. Focusing on ways that you can make your face appear happy, just may actually make you feel happy.

The next thing that I make a priority during my daily practice is to physically touch my patients. In our world today with cell phones, iPads and Facebook, many experts say we're craving the very thing that makes us such intelligent beings and that is real connection. One of the biggest ways you can connect with your patients is to lay your hands on them. I'm talking about the little gestures that show you are physically present and care.

Touch your patient's shoulder as they tell you they need something for pain. They are going to ask you for pain medicine anyway, so why not make them feel special by taking the NET experience and adding your hand to the mixture? Or the patient who you just helped to the bedside commode, tell him that you're just behind the curtain and at the same time place your hand warmly on his back.

As you start an IV, make sure you place your hand on the patient's arm while explaining the necessity of this painful experience. Touching each other connects us as humans we were created to be and are craving to return to. It also is one of the biggest factors that will make up the 55% of our body language communication approach.

I wish this could go without saying, but please make sure your physical touches are appropriate and just the right amount, not too much or too little. Always watch your patient's response to these gestures. And, of course, take into consideration different cultural beliefs when carrying out this form of communication. I love focusing on the shoulders, back and arms. These places are very accessible and touching there can rarely can be seen as inappropriate.

Remember, however, that when you are changing bed-bound patients, especially one who is alert and oriented, that this can be a very humiliating experience for them. In many cases, if I'm changing someone, I may touch their leg and politely ask them permission to turn or change them. Even though this may be an embarrassing experience, this gesture may make them feel more comfortable with you.

Touching is really effective when you have experiences where your attention is diverted elsewhere. How many times will your conversation be interrupted with the phone ringing or someone calling your name... all the time, right? When I'm in deep conversation with my patient or their loved ones and I'm interrupted, I simply place my hand on their shoulder and apologize as I answer the telephone or respond to the person.

The third personal behavior that you want to watch is to make sure you are making eye contact with your patients and their loved ones. Nothing says that you matter more than when someone looks into your eyes. Your patients and their family members are going to ask you questions and for things, and make sure you use your NET time again and glance their way.

When considering smiling, touching and eye contact, you may think you have all of this 55% part of communication covered. But there is another major factor that you need to watch, and that's your body. One day I was watching TV and there was a woman (I have totally forgotten her name and which channel it was even on) predicting whether celebrity couples were about to get divorced or not.

She was incredibly accurate in the past in predicting who and even when a couple was facing marital problems. On this show, she shared her very simple secret. She said that when looking at a picture of a couple, try to block out everything in the photo except the main direction in which the trunk of the person's body was facing and leaning.

If their trunks were kind of leaning into each other or facing each other, then their marriage was good. If however, they were even slightly leaning or facing the opposite directions, they were in trouble. Using this knowledge, I make an effort to make sure that the trunk of my body is facing and slightly leaning into whomever I am talking to. This way I'll show them that I am interested in the conversation and committed to understanding the message they are trying to give me.

The fifth and final factor that I wanted to mention in this chapter is breathing. As you learned in anatomy and physiology, breathing is one of the body's most important vehicles for moving waste material out of the body. In our every day lives, the stress we endure can make it natural for us to breathe very shallow breaths. These shallow breaths use only a fraction of our lung capacity and with the build up of toxins, can make us feel even more stressed.

Caroline Porter Thomas

What we must do is to consciously make an effort to take deep breaths as we go about our day. One of the best things I ever did was take a yoga class. I wouldn't say I'm a regular, but I do try to go three to four times a month. What these classes teach though is how to incorporate breathing into your daily movements. The instructor will advise you to move your leg to your right while taking a nice deep breath and then bend all the way down while letting the breath out slowly.

You can make triggers for yourself at work to help you remember to take these vital deep breaths. One thing I've done is to use triggers that used to stress me out to now remind me to take a deep breath. For example, I used to freak out every time my phone would ring… imagine how many times a day I freaked out? So I said to myself, "Every time the phone rings, I will be reminded to take a nice deep breath."

It also used to stress me out when I had to walk up and down, up and down the very long hallways. So I said to myself, "Every time I see a long hallway, I will be challenged to breathe in the entire length." These practices help me answer the phone with a sound mind and feel revitalized after finishing the length of the long hallway. Think of the things you encounter every day and let those experiences be triggers for you to remember to take the life-giving deep breaths.

The last topic I wanted to talk about in this communication chapter is how to connect with your patients and their loved ones who do not speak the same language as you. Of course, all hospitals have language lines via the telephone to help you exchange the verbal content of the message. Sometimes, however, I know there are simple requests that your patients or family members won't want to go through the five-minute system to ask for something little.

Many times with these little requests I see nurses get frustrated because they don't "speak" the same language. Living in Miami, Fla., I hear nurses say, "My patient doesn't like me because I don't speak Spanish." Although this may be true, I've found that that using my 93% of non-verbal communication can build deep connections with my patients using almost no words at all.

Always remember that as human beings we all share similar bodies. A facial expression of happiness is the same in every culture. The tonality, arm movements and body postures are also the same. Many times without words, only by watching your patient, you can find out that they would like more water, or that they need a towel or toothbrush. For these patients, your goal is to focus more intensely on using the 93% of communication.

And you will soon find that words really are a measly 7% of how we humans connect.

Caroline Porter Thomas

Chapter 15

How to Turn Around Complaints

"God grant me the serenity to accept the things I cannot change, the courage to change the things I can, and the wisdom to know the difference." – Reinhold Niebuhr

I was in the middle of report when another nurse ran up to me and interrupted us. "I have to give you one patient as soon as possible. I really need to go home to take my kids to school and if the patient's son shows up, I'm stuck here." Oh boy, I thought, not a good sign. I finished report with the other nurse quickly and then went to speak to this nurse.

"The patient is fine; she is here for failure to thrive and dehydration. She is 98 years old and it is very obvious that she wants to go on from this world." I glanced at the patient as we were in the room. The patient did have a gloomy and stressed out look on her face. "She is non-verbal, but she'll groan when you turn or clean her. She really just wants to be left alone." She continued the report, explaining that the woman was on IV fluids, but had placed in her will that she didn't want a feeding tube.

Her review of the systems also didn't look promising. Neuro wise, the patient wasn't responding to even her name. She was blind and deaf, per her son. Her lungs were hard to hear because she was so tiny and breathed shallowly; she was A-fib on the cardiac monitor (which is an irregular rhythm that can be managed with medical therapy).

The doctors ordered a Foley catheter due to incontinence and a very large sacral decubitis. It was unknown when her last bowel movement was due to her arrival two days prior and no one recollected from the nursing home. Musculoskeletal report showed her arms and legs were completely contracted. In addition to the one bed sore on her sacrum, she had five more scattered throughout her body. My heart really went out to her.

"The problem is the son," the nurse continued. "He comes in early every day, yelling at the nurses, doctors and calling administration saying that we have practically killed her." She is 98, I thought, and just looking at her I could tell none of this happened in two days. "He is completely irrational," the nurse said. I guess she read my mind.

"Just make sure she is turned exactly every 2 hours and I mean to the minute..." My mind was starting to think of all my other patients as she continued a very long list of things to do that the son wanted. Today I had six other patients and a few of them were extremely ill and would require a lot of nursing care. I was beginning to feel overwhelmed. I said a quiet prayer to myself. "God, please let this son be nice and calm today."

As I began my day, I worked with the nursing assistant and by 9 a.m. we were ahead of the game. We had already turned our lady twice and given her a nice bath. We combed her hair, brushed her teeth as best we could and changed all of her dressings. Both of us tried to feed her, but we weren't able to get a good amount of food in her. She kept spitting it out.

Somehow since we were moving so quickly and efficiently I was also able to keep up with my other patients as well. This is really impressive considering the huge amount of work seven patients can be. I had already assessed and documented on four of my seven patients and was also able to give all of my 8 a.m. meds. I was pushing myself to stay focused and efficient and it was working.

I was in a room a few doors down from my little lady's when… I heard him. I didn't hear him complain, yell or even speak. All I heard was the intense and very loud thud on the ground as he walked down the hall. I looked up from my other patient's room and thought back to my prayer… it hadn't seemed to work. But God and I have a relationship and I know that many times he doesn't give me what I want. He gives me what I need, and that day I guess I needed a lesson…

From my other patient's room I heard the call bell go on as soon as he stepped in. The bell was answered by the unit secretary and she asked what he needed. "Send my nurse in now," was all he said. What else could he want? I thought. Does he have any idea the amount of work I have done for his mother? How could he possibly be upset?

I went in the room and was greeted by his cold, stern face. He wasn't a large man, maybe 5'8", but his presence was huge; he moved his arms and hands in quick and abrupt patterns, he leaned his face to one side and with fire in his eyes peered into my eyes as he walked around his mother lifting the sheets and examining her every body part.

"Mr. Smith, how can I help you?" I asked, hoping that after examining her he would realize that we had given the best nursing care.

"I want the name of every single doctor, nurse and case manager who has been assigned to her care!" This question really caught me by surprise. A million thoughts were going through my mind, and I was wondering how I would be able to get the name of every single person who had taken care of her for the last two days. Right then I pictured myself sitting in the courtroom with him yelling at me in the judge's presence, his arms even more animated as he accused me of being a bad nurse.

"Become present," I said to myself. When I was in nursing school, I would become overwhelmed with stress

and my mind would quickly go to worst case scenario.
These images would be so scary and have such power over
me that sometimes I would become almost paralyzed and
not be able to take any action at all. Luckily I read this
great book by Paulo Coelho called *The Alchemist*. This
book is about a shepherd boy who tries to realize his
personal legend by following his heart.

He meets a very wise man who understands his
dream and helps him along the way. During the journey
there were many times the shepherd boy is scared and sees
himself unable to make his dream come true. One time he
expressed to the old wise man that his heart was scared of
this failure. The wise man responded, "Tell your heart that
the fear of suffering is worse than the suffering itself and
that no heart has ever suffered when it goes in search of its
dream... because every second of the search is a second
encounter with God and Eternity."

So while trying to focus and having fearful thoughts
creep in, I would realize that this fear is much worse than it
would actually be if I did fail. I found a way out of this
fear and it was to become present in this moment, in this
location. I'd take a deep breath and notice all of the things
around me. This would take me out of this scary future and
back into the present moment. I looked at the things
around me, the desk, table, kitchen, my books and I would
be grateful for this present moment.

With this feeling of gratitude, I would be able to see
a different vision. I would see myself as having achieved
the goal and project myself into a future that excited me.
These visions were and still are so powerful that I would
feel like I was zapped with energy and ready to take on the
task at hand.

I stood in the room with this man peering into my
soul. I noticed that his eyes were pale blue and hurting. I
noticed that his shoulders were flexed, but tired. I noticed
the room was warm and the bedside table could be cleaned

off. In this present moment, I gave thanks for the opportunity to be here. I then asked for guidance from this powerful presence that I was giving thanks to.

"Sir, I don't know how to get that information for you. Later I will be more than happy to ask my charge nurse to assist me. But sir, what can I do for you and your mother right now?" My voice was soft, a huge contrast from his harsh and loud tone. As I said this to him, in my imagination I saw his eyes sparkle with life and a smile form across his face.

"Well, let's at least turn her," he replied, his voice much different, soft and lower. It had not even been 45 minutes since we last turned her, but I didn't dare mention that to him. "Of course," I said, "let me just call for some help." After the nursing assistant and I turned her, he seemed satisfied.

"You know, three years ago we were traveling together." A smile came across his face as he looked up. You could see the happy memories coming back to him. In my head I was thinking in disbelief… she would have been 95 years old! "That is really amazing! She must have loved traveling with you!" For a few minutes, he told me where they had gone and how he had taken his 95-year-old mother on these journeys. Then my phone rang and I had to go and do something else.

I was a little behind, but with focusing and moving very fast I was able to stay on track. I gave each of my patients the very best care that I was capable of and it seemed to be paying off. I was pushing myself and imagining that I was a peak performance athlete and that I needed to stay focused, breathe deep and stay hydrated so that I could win the race… the race was staying caught up.

Every time I went in her room to turn her or to give a medication, he would tell me about some of their travels. I think that it had been a long time since he let himself recall the time that his mother and he enjoyed together. I was just delighted hearing how long life can be and that even into your 90's you can still have a lot of traveling ahead of you. We laughed together, and I literally almost cried hearing all of the wonderful stories of my little lady. I truly enjoyed my time that day with my patient and his son.

I couldn't help but think of how that day could have gone. What if when he first came to me demanding the names of the nurses and doctors I had gone straight to get the charge nurse? I could have easily said to the charge nurse, "Listen, I have seven patients and no time to deal with this son." I would have had a point and it really was true.

From experiences in the past, however, I've learned it's better to first do everything you can to handle the situation yourself. You see it takes just as much time trying to track down the charge nurse and update her of the situation, than it does to just see what you can do in that moment. Also, when you will be updating the charge nurse you will most likely be emotionally charged in a negative way and this feeling can make it hard for you to get any of your work done in that emotional state.

I finished that day with much more energy than I came with. I worked hard, moved fast and ate just enough to give me energy and stopped before the extra food would make me sleepy. I focused intently on how to deliver the best care in the most timely, efficient way.

When it came to my interactions with my co-workers and charge nurse, I didn't dare mention what had happened in the morning. The charge nurse had been notified by the previous night charge nurse that the son had multiple complaints and she asked me if I was ok. I told her I was. I know that whatever I think about or talk about, I will relive. Although it was a rough start in the morning, that is not what I wanted my lasting memories to be of my patient and her son.

Amazingly, I didn't even remember that he had asked me for the doctors' and nurses' names until I was in my car driving home. I couldn't help but laugh as I realized the power of stepping up and handling complaints. I know that God was teaching me that day that I can turn any complaint around; I just have to find the resources that are already inside each of us and trust that there is a way.

Caroline Porter Thomas

Chapter 16

How to Deal With Mistakes

"Mistakes are the usual bridge between inexperience and wisdom." – Phyllis Therous

"Forgive yourself for your faults and your mistakes and move on." – Les Brown

"The path to wisdom is not being afraid to make mistakes." – Paulo Coelho

When I was in nursing school, I was constantly reminded of nurses who lost their licenses due to the terrible mistakes they made. The professors would tell us constantly how people's lives were in our hands and that one small mistake on our part could have unthinkably terrible consequences to our patients. They would play movies of people talking about the mistakes that nurses made, and they would speak from their own experience of mistakes that they had seen or made themselves.

By the time I graduated nursing school, I was scared to death to give any medications or perform nursing tasks. Due to this fear, I clearly remember the very first medication that I gave. Before I passed the NCLEX examination, I was hired as a nursing assistant to shadow a nurse on the unit. This was a great experience because, since I did not have a license yet, I was really expected to just watch and learn.

Caroline Porter Thomas

The day after I passed the NCLEX examination and my title was changed from Nursing Assistant to Registered Nurse, I was more scared than ever to go to work due to this fear. I remember the exact moment where my preceptor thought it was a good time for me to administer my first medication. It was Tylenol... I know she had a lot of faith in me to start out with this critical medication.

Believe it or not, I really resisted giving this over–the-counter medication. I was so freaked out, I kept looking at the nursing drug guide, checking my patient's labs and then their vital signs. She finally placed her hand on my shoulder and said, "You're a Registered Nurse now, you can give this. This patient is able to have the Tylenol, go ahead and give it." Her tone suggested slight urgency because we had a lot of other things that we needed to do at that time too.

"Ok, ok, I got this," I said to myself. My eyes were wide open, my hands were shaking and I was walking into my room repeating the 5, 6 or now probably 11 rights to giving medication as if it was a prayer. It probably took me 10 minutes to give the Tylenol... but it was a success! Crazy, huh, how fear can have such control of us?

I know this fear is well founded. Many, many people have been hurt and, unfortunately, even killed by nursing mistakes. These nurses were probably really good people just like you and me; the only problem was that they made a mistake that cost them and others severely. The thought of working so hard for a nursing license and having the possibility of having it taken away is so painful. However, it is rare, but it does happen.

How do you deal with this fear of making a mistake? What I have found is that this fear is ultimately a good thing. It helps me focus a great deal on every task or medication that is ordered. Fear is a powerful force, and it can be used intelligently to help you become a great nurse. Every day that I am at work, while giving medications, I examine each medication and think of the worst-case scenario. I then examine my patient and run through a checklist -- what are their vital signs, what are their labs, what was their last blood sugar, what does this medication affect and what could go terribly wrong if given and it had a negative effect? Here is what I do after that step, and mind you, I only see the worst-case scenario for a second. Then I think about why it was ordered and the therapeutic benefits that it has on my patient. I also look to see whether this is the first time the patient is getting the medication. If my patient was admitted last shift and I am giving them all of their medications for the first time in the hospital, I am a lot more cautious.

You see, even if the doctor ordered all of the medications that the patient takes every day, we give almost all of those medications at the same time. So as you're going over the medications with your patient, explain the way the hospital schedules the medications and ask them if they have ever taken them this way. Sometimes the patient will be on multiple blood pressure medications and they will say, "I take this one in the morning and that one in the evening."

If a doctor orders a medication to be given "daily," the pharmacy automatically selects a time based on the medication and the normal administration time. In the example above, you can call pharmacy and ask them to change the time for that particular medication so your patient can stay on schedule. Helping your patients stay on their regimen can help their body focus on getting better.

All of this seems like a lot of work, and really it is, especially at first. What does help though is that when you are working on a particular unit you give a lot of the same medications over and over so this process becomes quicker over time. Really, the more you work, the easier it becomes. I had one older, wise nurse tell me on my first job that, "We do the same things over and over; the only problem is that we do lots and lots of tasks, but still it really is the same things over and over."

What I have also found is that you will make mistakes. Every nurse does. Especially in units where you have six or seven patients or maybe in a specialty unit where you have a lot going on with your patients and are having a hard time keeping up. In this chapter, I want to walk you through some of my major mistakes. What I have found is that you can learn a great deal from other people's experiences, both good and bad.

My first error was the classic, giving the wrong medication to the wrong patient. Of course, I remember that day as if it was yesterday. It was my last day of orientation and I really wanted to show my preceptor and the director of the unit that I had been trained well and was ready to take a full patient load on my own. As I was getting report, I was pumping myself up and finding ways I could be super efficient and super fast.

After report, I started my assessments and medications. I went into the first room, checked her vital signs and went through each medication with the patient as I usually do. I was carful to examine each medication and was talking to her the entire time. We got deep into a conversation and then suddenly she looked at me and said, "Honey, I know you're busy. Give me the medications so you can go to your next patients." I did just that and she took them.

Before I left, she asked if I could bring her a pair of socks. As I was leaving the room another nurse on the unit saw me and gave me a puzzled look and then asked me if the patient needed anything. "She asked for socks." I was a little puzzled, too, that the nurse asked me that. It didn't register immediately. I began to get medications for another patient but inside my head that question came up again, "Why did she ask me what my patient wanted?"

Then my heart sank. I looked at my assignment, I looked at the chart (we did paper charting then) and then I ran out and looked at the room. "Oh my God, oh my God, what do I do???" I quickly mentally retraced my steps of giving the medications and realized that I forgot to check my patient's arm band! I was shaking when I went over to the nurse who obviously was assigned to that patient. "Ummm, I don't know what to do... I just gave your patient one of my patient's medications.

She looked at me in disbelief, but then quickly awoke from that state. "Let me see the medications that you gave." I went over and grabbed the chart as we looked at exactly what I gave the woman. We examined both of the lists side by side to see what medications were different and similar. She helped me write down the wrong and potentially dangerous medications that I had given to report to the doctor and instructed me to take frequent vital signs and watch the patient closely.

I notified the doctor, who was a bit annoyed, but understanding. He gave new instructions on how to adjust the patient's medications for the day as well as how often to monitor. Thankfully, everything worked out, and the patient was fine; her vital signs never really fluctuated and she was very understanding of my mistake. She even hugged me when we finished talking.

Another thing that was amazing was that all of the experienced nurses who came around to offer me words of encouragement. They spoke of the mistakes they had personally made and of mistakes they had seen. What I quickly realized was that from making one mistake, I really learned a lot from other people's mistakes.

Because I have been a nurse for five years, that is a lot of time to make even more mistakes. Just so you can learn a little more from me, I want to share with you a few more. Another big mistake that I made was with the medication Cardizem. The doctor ordered my patient to receive this medication every eight hours. So at 2 p.m. it was scheduled. This time I had everything right, the right medication, right patient, right dose...

I quickly glanced at my patient's blood pressure and it was fine 143/72 or something close to that. I gave her the medication and went on with my day. About an hour later, I was in the room while the nursing assistant was taking her vital signs. "I feel dizzy," the patient said. Hmmm, I thought, why would she feel dizzy? I also began to look at her closely, seeing she had a few sweat bubbles forming on her forehead.

"Hey, Caroline, look." The nursing assistant pointed at her heart rate, which was in the low 40's and high 30's. My eyes got wide and I asked the assistant, "What should I do???" She responded, "I think you should get help." Holy cow, that is exactly what I need to do. I love how smart my nursing assistants are sometimes. I called the charge nurse and told her that I needed help.

She asked me why and what was going on. "Well, my patient says she is feeling dizzy, her heart rate is in the high 30's low 40's and she is diaphoretic." That was all she needed to hear and she was there in a split second. A few other nurses came to help out and we started examining what was going on. "Caroline, her heart rate was 47 when you gave the Cardizem."

Oh wow, I thought as I realized that I looked at my patient's blood pressure, but completely forgot Cardizem is a medication that is mainly to help control the heart rate. Literally, I started to cry; it wasn't pretty. The patient's doctor happened to be on the floor and was called to the room. Atropine had to be given in order to increase her heart rate and she was transferred to the ICU for closer monitoring.

This entire time, I was having a hard time keeping myself from crying. Even as I gave report to the ICU nurse, I was tearing up. The patient was stable before we transferred her. Her heart rate was up to the 50's and her dizziness was gone. So thank God there were no long-term consequences for my mistake. As I left the ICU, the nurse stopped me. "Caroline, it is ok, you are human and mistakes like this are made every day." She hugged me and told me that this would just make me a better nurse.

Since then, of course, I've made plenty more mistakes. One day at 11:30, my patient's blood sugar flashed up as a new result in the Meditech system and said her blood glucose was 430. "Again?" I thought as the nurse before me had said that his blood sugar had been in the 400's for the morning and she had covered him for it. So when lunch arrived, I gave him the proper amount of fast-acting insulin. As I was leaving the room, I noticed that on the board the nursing assistant had written 239.

Since I float to multiple hospitals and units, I was not familiar with this unit's system of the nursing assistant writing the blood sugars results on the patient's white board. "Uh oh," I thought as I quickly logged in to glance at that result again. As I looked at it, I noticed that the result at 430 had been taken at 0700. "Oh, my God," I thought. I quickly ran and grabbed the glucometer and rechecked the result. It was still high in the 300's but that could quickly change with the amount of insulin I had given.

I called the doctor, who had a few words to say about my mistake, but ultimately ordered me to give IV D50 and monitor the blood sugar frequently. I did just that and the patient remained stable, with his blood sugars never going below the 200's. To this day I have no idea why it flashed up as a new result at 1130, but I learned a lesson the hard way that day. I now examine the times very closely.

The last mistake I will share is this. You do have to question the doctor's orders if they don't make sense. I received a patient who the doctor admitted for possible appendicitis. The doctor wrote a page of orders. The very first medication at the top of the sheet he wrote for 40mg of Lovenox sub-q STAT. On the lower end of the sheet, he wrote a consultation for the surgeon.

Realizing that that was a weird combo of orders, I did some brief questioning in my head. Why would the Lovenox be ordered near the top of the orders and why STAT? If the Lovenox was ordered STAT then the doctor must suspect a blood clot of some kind. I gave the medication as quickly as I could.

About two hours later, my charge nurse informed me that they wanted to take the patient to the operating room at that second. I wasn't to worry about the paperwork, they would complete it right then. "Surgery now? I just gave the patient Lovenox!?" She instructed me to write a note for the OR nurse and place it on the chart. I did that.

The next day I went into work and the director of the unit asked to speak with me immediately. As I was talking to her, she explained that the surgeon was never informed that the patient had Lovenox and that they had done the surgery and the patient lost a lot of blood. The patient was fine and her H&H never dropped below 10 & 28; however, to be cautious, the patient had to be transferred to the ICU for closer monitoring. She also told me that the patient did receive a transfusion due to the loss of blood.

We went over what had happened that day and I realized that my first instinct was correct. I should have called the doctor and asked why the STAT Lovenox as well as the surgical consult? I also learned that I should have verbally told the surgeon that I had given Lovenox, as maybe some vitamin K could have been given to prevent this complication. Thank God this patient was stable and ultimately made a full recovery, but it just shows that doctors write weird orders sometimes. If it doesn't feel right, trust your gut and give them a clarification call.

I want you to notice something. I've made these mistakes as well as many more. Every nurse does and you will, as well. The main piece of advice I can offer you is to get in the habit of looking at the big picture. Ninety-nine percent of mistakes are really not a big deal and can be managed with a little bit of effort.

I also want to encourage you to connect with your creator – whatever your beliefs are -- frequently while you are at work. You need to understand that everything happens for a reason, although many times we don't know why because we are unable to see the whole picture. But having faith will help you remember that each of us is a small part of a big picture. That each of us really is a good person and we are doing the absolute best we can. And each action done right and each mistake made will only make us better nurses and people.

Caroline Porter Thomas

Chapter 17

How to Accept Your Patient's Passing

"Everything science has taught me—and continues to teach me—strengthens my belief in the continuity of our spiritual existence after death. Nothing disappears without a trace."
—*Wernher Von Braun*

"Consciousness is eternal it is not vanquished with the destruction of the temporary body."
— *Bhagavad Gita*

I clearly remember my first patient who died on my shift, under my care. This gentleman was in his 80's and had tertiary syphilis, which he had never sought treatment for. When I received him as a patient, he was unable to communicate properly. Most of his language was mumbling of sound with no words; every now and then, an English word would emerge but seemed to have no link to the conversation. His movements also would be in a frequent jerking fashion, mostly of the arms. Syphilis had affected his brain and spinal cord permanently.

His wife was at the bedside, a very warm, sweet and loving woman. She had been caring for her husband for the last few years as his condition deteriorated. I see caregivers all of the time and many of them are worn out and fed up. A lot of the times, once their loved one is admitted to the hospital, they go home to get some much needed respite time. I never really blame those individuals. Being a primary caregiver is a full-time job with few rewards, and many times I don't know how they do it.

This woman was different, though. She was happy and peaceful; she served her husband in the hospital with joy. When it was time to bathe the patient, she helped place the clean pillow cases on the pillows. We had to ask her to step aside as we pulled him up in bed because I couldn't see this 80-year-old woman help those of us in our 20's pull him up.

It was obvious to me that she served her husband with joy and honesty despite the obvious fact that the reason he was sick was from unfaithfulness due to his illness from a sexually transmitted disease. Anyone could see she still loved him. Even though she had that warm smile and quick readiness to serve at the drop of the hat, I could see that physically she was tired. I spoke with her in great length and convinced her that I would take really good care of her husband and that she could go home and sleep in her own bed.

I was working the 7 p.m. to 7 a.m. shift that night and she left the room at 9:30, kissing her husband on the head. I didn't think that much about her husband for a while. I was definitely busy with all of my patients and tons of paperwork and documenting that needed to be done. At about midnight, though, something changed with this man. The change was subtle and I really couldn't put my finger on it, but I could tell something was happening.

The color in his body was different, he was more quiet and less jerky. Hmmm, I thought, what is going on? I went to an experienced nurse, since I was new and had only been off orientation for about three months. She came and took a look at the patient and agreed that he didn't look that great. She instructed me to grab the vital sign machine and we could go from there.

I did just that, taking his blood pressure, heart rate, oxygen saturation and temperature. Everything was fine. BP was slightly elevated in the high 140's over 80's, but that had been his norm. I was sure his oxygen saturation was going to be low due to the slight change in the patient's color, but this, too, was fine, at 98%. Still I kept looking at him wondering what was going on; deep down I knew that something was going to happen.

Two hours later I got a call from the telemetry technician. "Caroline, your patient in room 343, his heart rate is dropping. It was in 80's now it's in the 50's… why don't you go check on him?" I got up immediately and began walking briskly to the room. I was halfway down the hallway with the technician still on my ear when she said, "His heart rate just dropped to 30!" I started to run.

When I reached the room I could tell that I needed to call a code blue immediately. My patient was lying in bed completely still and had his eyes open with a blank stare on them. His color now was even worse, very gray and ashen. "Oh no!" I thought. He looked as if he was dying, and I had convinced his wife that I would take care of him!

From this point on a flood of people from all over the hospital came in the room and began asking me what was going on. I told them his history and the situation as best I could. I was emotionally barely able to pull it together. I could tell this man wasn't breathing and one of the ICU nurses started CPR. Drugs were being administered, CPR was being continued and shocks were administered. Nothing was working. After about 20 minutes, the doctor on call who had come to the code, called it. Time of death was 0230.

"I need the number to his next of kin," the doctor said to me. "That would be his wife. I'll find her number." I told him as I walked over to the chart, feeling absolutely terrible about the news that she was about to hear and how I had failed her. The doctor took the number and went over in the corner and called the number. I tried to listen to the conversation, but the room was still noisy due to so many people being there.

"She will be here in about 20 minutes," he said. He signed a few pieces of paper that the nursing supervisor told him to sign and then was on his way. Twenty minutes, I thought, what do I need to do to get ready for her?

"Is this your first patient who ever died?" a woman's voice said to me. I looked over to find the same ICU nurse who had started the CPR. "Yes." At that point the room was very quiet; everyone had left and I was amazed how there was just me and this ICU nurse.

"I'll help you," she said. She was like my angel; she told me what I needed to do to get the body ready for the family. Together we removed all of the IV's and equipment that was attached to him. We cleaned him up and placed fresh, clean linen everywhere. She even helped me comb his hair and place some cologne that was in his room. We made his body look as dignified as possible.

By the time the family came, I decided that I was as ready as I ever would be. I was still dreading the look I would receive from his wife's eyes, but there really was nothing else I could do. The ICU nurse gave me a few more final instructions, hugged me, told me that I did everything I could and then went back to her unit. I learned a lot from her that day. She didn't have to stay; she could have left like everyone else. Why she decided to was beyond me. Not even people from my own unit, whom I considered my friends, were there with me. She gave me, and now you, a great example and I will be forever grateful for that. My real only regret was that I never got her name.

When she left, I suddenly realized that I was in a room alone with a dead person. Seriously, I had never seen anyone pass before and it is definitely a different feeling. I stood there for a minute and stared at my patient, amazed at the contrast of how he had been earlier when he was full of life and how he was now. Wow, this is where we all end up, I thought, and for a brief moment I contemplated what life was all about. I also began questioning why this happened, why this city, why this hospital and why in this bed that I was assigned to?

I didn't have long before the wife arrived with her son. She did look sad as I expected. But she also looked stronger than I remembered. She went over to her husband and placed her hand on his forehead and said a silent prayer and cried. I had been holding back tears all night, but at this moment I also started to cry. When she looked up at me and saw me crying, she held out her other hand for me to hold and I stood there with her for just a minute.

She told me that God was in charge of everything and that this was His will. She also thanked me for taking such good care of him. Good care? I thought... did you forget that your husband died under my care? "My husband has been sick for a long time," she said. "I knew this was coming and I'm thankful that it was with you." I thought about that for a long time after she left.

I watched this video from Steve Jobs, a commencement speech to the graduates from Stanford University. He bluntly spoke of death and how it is possibly the single greatest invention since life. I realized that the meaning you give to someone's passing on makes all the difference.

Initially I blamed myself for my patient's passing. I questioned what if I had just called the doctor and said that this patient doesn't look right. Maybe something would have been different. Maybe if I had checked on him more frequently this wouldn't have happened. What if I didn't convince his wife to leave? I carried all of these thoughts in my head and they literally weighed me down.

I realized that my outlook on death was something that I created in my imagination using only my senses. I would imagine a dead body that would soon be rotting and smell terrible. Eventually it would just be bones. I was shutting out the fact that I know more exists than this life because I feel it. I then changed the vision in my head and now feel so much more at peace with my patient's passing, and even with my own impending demise.

As a nurse, you will come in closer proximity to death when compared to other career fields. There are obviously specialties that will see more and some that will see less of it. If you work in a Pediatric ICU you could see very young people die. If you work on an oncology unit, you may also see a lot of people pass. There are units where it is rare, such as the Mother/Baby units.

What I have realized is that the main factor that influences your feelings about death is the vision you have created about it. We all have different beliefs about the meaning of life and death. What I want you to understand, though, is that this is something you create. Your culture, religion and upbringing most of the time build this blueprint, but you are the artist with the last say.

I encourage you to design a vision of what death means that will empower you. Maybe this means that we all go to heaven, walk with Jesus or pass on to another body in another life. Whatever the case, make sure it's something that moves you and helps you give great care to all of your patients, especially those who are close or have passed. I personally like the words of Mother Teresa "Let us touch the dying, the poor, the lonely and the unwanted according to the graces we have received and let us not be ashamed or slow to do the humble work."

Chapter 18

How to LOVE Your
First Job as a Nurse!

"A vision keeps the wealthy soul focused on the path and not the boulders." – Michael Northwood

"Growth means change and change involves risk, stepping from the known to the unknown." – Benjamin Franklin

I remember one day when I was fairly new to being a nurse. I was feeling overwhelmed at the time and had a good 10 important tasks that all needed to be done "now." As the rest of my co-workers and charge nurse also appeared flustered, I felt as if I had no one to ask for help. So I powered through my to-do list as best I could, prioritizing and re-prioritizing constantly. I finally got to a point where I didn't feel like I could handle my load and asked one of the nurses on the unit for a hand.

"I can't," was all this nurse said as she ran off as soon as possible. I stood there for a moment understanding that I didn't have the time to be mad at her. I really did need to page a doctor concerning my patient's high blood pressure. When the doctor called back, his voice was rough and abrupt. He gave me an order for a medication I'd never heard of.

This doctor had a very heavy accent that didn't help matters. "I'm sorry, could you repeat that?" I asked him. Again he said something in a very heavy accent. Only this time he was so loud that the voice over the phone was sort of fuzzy… which of course only meant that I really couldn't understand the order. After that, he asked me to put someone on the phone who knew what they were doing.

Later that day, things didn't improve. I went into one of my patient's rooms only to be greeted by her entire family with folded arms and less than friendly looks on their face. "Why have you been withholding pain medicine from my mom?!?" one of them shouted at me. Their mother had unfortunately suffered from a stroke and was unable to communicate verbally. She did make facial movements and could slightly squeeze her right hand on demand. I hadn't noticed any signs that she was in pain.

"I'm so sorry," I said, really not understanding why they thought she was in pain. She looked quite comfortable to me. "How do you know she is in pain?" He looked at me again the same way. "Can you read?" I didn't answer but just looked around for something that I should have read earlier. There was a sign above their mother's bed that read "One squeeze of the right hand is yes and two is no." Oh yea, I thought. The night nurse did say that in report.

At this moment, I felt like all of my thoughts were blurry. All I could hear was all of the disappointments from earlier today, which included but were certainly not limited to the nurse who had refused to help me earlier and the doctor with the heavy accent who asked to speak to someone else. "What's going on?" I said to myself, wondering why I had such lack of control with my thought process.

I glanced around and noticed that the TV in the patient's room was very loud and Judge Judy was on. "Do you mind if I turn the TV off?" I said to my patient's family members. Puzzled by my question, he told me that was fine. Wow… what a difference! My mind felt almost completely clear. I took a deep breath and looked into the options that I had to help their mother.

Once I had satisfied this family's needs and gave their mother the medication they suggested, I asked myself.

"What else can I do to make this a POWERFUL DAY?!?" This question is one of the best tools I can give you. I can't tell you how valuable it is. It is this question ALONE, I believe, that gives me the power to correct any wrong and turn any terrible day into the best day ever! You see, regardless of what you believe religiously you must admit that there must be some wisdom in the Bible, for it to still be around today. "Seek and Ye Shall Find."

I evaluated my thought process from earlier. What had been going through my mind? I'd been looking at what seemed to be the mountain of things that needed to be done and only had a fuzzy brain to work with. First of all, I was in a very loud and hectic environment. You can't control all of the sounds, but you can minimize your exposure.

One of the things that I had been doing was going into my patient's rooms to perform tasks or give medications. When I was finished, I left the room and went into the hallway or the nurse's area to think about my next task. Well, the hallway and the nurse's area were some of the loudest and most chaotic places to be. Most of my patients' rooms were much quieter. I began to stay one extra minute in my patients' rooms as I planned my next action. Of course, not every single patient's room was a quiet and great place to think. But I would venture to say that 90% of the rooms will grant you a minute of clear thinking.

"What else can I do?" I thought. I noticed that just like in the scenario earlier, when my patients had the TV on very loud it affected my thinking. I got in the habit of asking if it was ok to turn the TV off for a minute so I could speak to them and give them my full attention. Ninety-nine percent of my patients were literally overjoyed to do this. Many times I would hear them say that they weren't watching it anyway. This also encouraged conversations with my patients and we got to know each other better.

"What else can I do?" Why had I gotten upset with the nurse who refused to help me and the doctor with the heavy accent? Is it possible that this nurse was having a worse day than me? Of course that is possible. I then chose to approach her as if nothing had ever happened and our relationship only got better. And the situation with the doctor – is it possible that I was the 20th nurse who asked him to repeat himself five times? Was it also possible that this doctor had an office full of patients needing to see him? I chose to treat him as if nothing had happened and our relationship also got better.

"What else can I do?" My thoughts then led me to examine the questions I had been asking myself earlier. What were the words that I was using that were making me feel fuzzy and powerless? I realized that I was asking the question "Why?" Why did I have so much work to do? Why did I have so many patients? Why would no one help me? Why do we have doctors who can't speak English? Why is my patient's blood pressure so high?

What is the difference in these questions? I was beginning to understand that the question of "Why?" had no empowering answer. Whereas the questions of, "What else can I do?" helped me think of ways to handle, do or turn around situations. One question empowered and one question paralyzed me. I created these questions in the first place, so I have the power as to which question I choose. I consciously choose now to ask the empowering question of "What else can I do?"

This question led me to pay special attention to my body and its needs. Many times before I go into a patient's room, the answer to this question leads me to have a very quick snack or take a quick bathroom break. This really helps, especially when you know you're going to be in the room for a while. This will help you approach the situation with a clear mind as opposed to dreaming about your next snack while your patient is talking to you.

Through the guidance of this question I have learned to be led by the mantra, "Feel good yourself first." I have learned on more than one occasion that it's harder to help your patient feel better when you don't feel good yourself. Notice that I did not say impossible, I just said that it is harder. Sometimes all your patient needs is a genuine smile or kind touch. I believe patients can tell the difference between a stressed show of teeth and a hurried touch, so I ask my favorite question and find out how I can have the former.

In my experience with life and now my experience in the hospital, I learned that you choose what you will see. In the untrained eye, this hospital can be a very negative, overwhelming and scary place when you ask why it is so. Why did you get this patient load? Why did this doctor order this procedure? Why does this patient's family member feel like they have to stay? The answers to these questions will all lead you to believe that this is a negative environment, literally blinding you to the good things that go on during the day.

It takes work and is a daily practice to choose to see the beauty that is already there. This is a process that I myself have to work on daily. If you have ever worked with me or know someone who has worked with me, you know that I am not exempt from this daily duty. I find myself at times reading my own words and realizing that I'm not practicing what I'm teaching. My only hope is to become better and better at this. The comfort that I do have, though, is that I have the tools I need to turn everything around and it is my prayer that you now feel the same.

Whether you hate your first job or love it depends on you. You choose daily what you want to focus on. You cannot be the best nurse to every patient every single time.

But were you an outstanding nurse to one patient today? Focus on that victory and you'll find that you will have the energy and power to be an outstanding nurse more often.

Asking the question "What else can I do?" will help you find ways to make your job doable and more enjoyable. Guys, my greatest dream is to reignite the love of nursing that led Florence Nightingale and many of the other amazing nurses who went before us. Please, if this book or my videos have touched you in any way, email me at Caroline@EmpoweRN.com and tell me. My dream one day is to meet you and have amazing conversations about how you love being a nurse and how you are such an asset to every patient you touch.

If this book has helped you in any way, please forward it to your friends and classmates. Believe me, nursing is about teamwork and the better the people around you are doing, the better your chances of success!

I look forward to hearing from you!

Until next time!

With Much Love,

-Caroline Porter Thomas

www.EmpoweRN.com

New Nurse? How to Get, Keep and LOVE Your First Job!

Caroline Porter Thomas